THE WOMAN WHO CRACKED
THE ANXIETY CODE

Judith Hoare is a journalist who worked for the
Australian Broadcasting Corporation and *The
Australian Financial Review*. She started her career on
Chequerboard, a trailblazing social-issues program in
the 1970s, and then moved to *AFR*, reporting on
federal politics in Canberra. She shifted to features
writing, to eventually specialise in editing long-form
journalism for the newspaper, and was appointed
deputy editor, features, in 1995, a position she held
for 20 years.

THE WOMAN
WHO CRACKED
THE ANXIETY
CODE

THE EXTRAORDINARY LIFE
OF DR CLAIRE WEEKES

Judith Hoare

SCRIBE
Melbourne • London

Scribe Publications
2 John Street, Clerkenwell, London, WC1N 2ES, United Kingdom
18–20 Edward St, Brunswick, Victoria 3056, Australia
3754 Pleasant Ave, Suite 100, Minneapolis, Minnesota 55409 USA

First published by Scribe 2019

Typeset in 12.5/17 pt Bembo Book MT Std by the publishers.

Printed and bound in the UK by CPI Group (UK) Ltd, Croydon CR0 4YY

Scribe Publications is committed to the sustainable use of natural resources and the
use of paper products made responsibly from those resources.

9781912854165 (UK edition)
9781950354108 (US edition)
9781925713381 (Australian edition)
9781925693751 (e-book)

Catalogue records for this book are available from the National Library of
Australia and the British Library.

scribepublications.co.uk
scribepublications.com
scribepublications.com.au

For Jim, Claudia, and Kate

The way we are living,
timorous or bold,
will have been our life.

Seamus Heaney

Contents

Prologue

THE UNCOMMON SENSE
OF CLAIRE WEEKES

On 23 October 1977, a diminutive Australian stepped onto the stage in New York. The audience saw an elderly woman whose regular uniform was a tweed skirt, twin-set, spectacles, and sensible brown lace-up shoes with low heels. Her dark hair was permed and for adornment she preferred a string of pearls.

At the age of 74, Dr Claire Weekes was the guest speaker at the 18th Annual Fall Conference of the Association for the Advancement of Psychotherapy. She was an unusual choice for this gathering as she ranked as an unqualified outsider.

However, Weekes had one measurable claim to fame: her books on anxiety were a global sensation, hitting bestseller lists in the US and the UK. She had found a popular audience by identifying and describing the havoc nervous illness could create and explaining and treating it in a fresh way. Weekes had been invited to address this professional association despite divided opinion over her approach. Many psychiatrists had heard of her methods from their patients, and a number accepted that some patients they had treated unsuccessfully had read her books and felt, if not entirely cured, then on the way to recovery.

Weekes had written the prosaically titled *Self Help for Your Nerves* in 1962, and, by the time she was standing on the podium in New York over 15 years later, there had been two more books, which were prominently displayed in airports and translated into at least eight languages. For years, the professionals had looked away from, and down on, her work.

The books were slim volumes that explained the nervous system and how it could go awry, how the mind and body were interconnected in arousal, and the trouble this could cause. Yet the clarity of work that drove the books' runaway success also repelled professional recognition. Self-help was not yet a genre that inspired psychiatrists' attention or respect.

Earlier that year, her third book, *Simple, Effective Treatment of Agoraphobia*, had been published in the US. It was her first directed at the medical community, and in it she asserted that far from helping their patients, psychoanalysts often made matters worse. She also corrected one of the pre-eminent British psychologists, Dr Isaac Marks, who put agoraphobia before anxiety. Weekes reversed the order, arguing that anxiety — or, more specifically, fear — came first, and triggered agoraphobia. The profession was on notice that she believed she had the answers to problems they were misconstruing.

As Weekes toured the US from coast to coast, she was interviewed by well-known television talk-show hosts, and countless newspaper articles were written about her work and syndicated across the country.

In a field more familiar with failure, and one riven with division, Weekes achieved success. Indeed, such was the confusion and disenchantment with the lack of progress in treating the mentally ill that in the 1970s a group of psychiatrists launched an 'anti-psychiatry' movement. Their manifesto proclaimed that rather than suffering from mental illness, their patients were victims of society.

Underneath it all was a growing unease with the lack of empirical evidence for any treatment, which invited the question of how to measure success or failure. Yet Weekes had the numbers running in her favour. People bought her books and queued to thank her for 'saving' their lives. She was writing about 'them'. Many chose a religious metaphor to express their gratitude. The books were their 'bible'.

On the podium in New York, Weekes inspired no awe and many in the audience dismissed her as a populist. That she was a medical practitioner and held a doctorate in science as well did not count. She was the author of self-help books, she was not a psychiatrist, and she was in huge demand in the media. Her fame invited critical attention to her lack of specialist credentials, which was enough to wound her reputation in her own profession.

She had one professional advocate, however — the New York psychiatrist Dr Manuel Zane. He had founded the first hospital-based phobia and anxiety clinic in the United States, at White Plains, New York, just six years earlier and had seen for himself how the Weekes method worked. Zane had been impressed by the heartfelt response to her books from a number of his own intractable patients, who had been housebound for years.

By the time Zane opened his clinic in 1971, Weekes was already a phenomenon in the field of anxiety. A clinician pioneering his own unorthodox method of treatment, he had an open mind, and saw some common ground in her approach.

He wrote to Weekes in Australia, inviting her to visit his clinic in New York. As a result of his passionate advocacy, she gained wider access to US mental-health professionals. Zane pressed upon his colleagues his view that Weekes had a special and unique understanding of anxiety, particularly panic disorder. Better still, she had an easily understood and demonstrably effective treatment protocol.

With the patronage of Zane among others, Weekes was invited from time to time to address professionals, but she felt their resistance, and some criticised her openly. During at least one of her public lectures, she was keenly aware that psychiatrists in the front row consulted their watches every few minutes. Others talked audibly to each other.

Her speech in New York in 1977 was an explicit challenge to the prevailing orthodoxies, and she was combative. She gave her address the same title as her latest book, 'Simple, Effective Treatment of Agoraphobia'.

In the audience were psychiatrists who fell into one of two schools. They were either psychoanalysts, who followed the techniques of Freud and his intellectual descendants, or cognitive behaviourists, who worked on changing habits of thought and associated behaviours. Both would have been provoked by her presentation.

If there were hackles raised generally, there was one individual who must have felt she was especially plucking his feathers. The renowned South African psychiatrist Dr Joseph Wolpe was a behaviourist who built a reputation for treating exactly the high-anxiety or panic states Weekes was talking about. She later confided to a colleague that Wolpe had 'torn her to pieces' that day.

Weekes and Wolpe could agree on one thing. Like Weekes, Wolpe rejected Freudian psychoanalysis and the obsession with unconscious drives rooted in childhood experiences, such as the Oedipus complex and others now common to everyday language.

Instead, Wolpe focused entirely on behaviour. His reputation for pioneering behavioural therapy was based on his early work scaring cats with electrical shocks. He then rewarded them with food in an effort to eradicate the neuroses he had created.

Moving from animals to humans, Wolpe encouraged exposure to phobias and fears, as patients were simultaneously taught to relax. He pioneered a strategy called desensitisation, which was otherwise known as exposure therapy. That is, anxious patients were taught how to face their particular fear while practising relaxation strategies.

Later, Weekes was also regarded as a 'pioneer' of so-called 'exposure therapy', yet never used the phrase herself and was not advocating relaxation but something quite different. She objected openly to the proposition that the highly anxious individual could or should be 'desensitised'. This was tackling the problem the wrong way around.

'Rather than aiming to adapt to difficult situations, to achieve desensitization by suggestions, or to avoid panic, the agoraphobe must learn to pass through panic and to rid oneself of drug dependency. This method of self-desensitization will, as a rule, achieve results quickly and does not necessarily depend upon finding the cause of the original sensitization,' she told the psychiatrists assembled in New York.

Trying to teach a patient to relax in the face of phobia or panic was not only counterproductive but an almost impossible mission. Instead, she argued that by fully experiencing the panic, the individual learned it was possible to 'pass through' to the other side. Their nervous system needed to be reordered, which they could learn to do themselves. They didn't then need a shepherd or psychiatrist.

Nervous illness was felt intensely in the body. In her book, she described 'the whiplash of panic' and the 'electrifying quality of sensitised panic' to communicate to a non-sufferer the way in which continued distress prepared the body to ever more swiftly respond. The nervous system became primed to experience anxiety more quickly and savagely than ever. It had become 'sensitised', and understanding this process was the key to recovery. Desensitisation would follow as a natural consequence. That is, there was no need to practise becoming desensitised to whatever was particularly feared.

So instead of structured exposure to fears, she prescribed total acceptance of the fear as the way out of distress and panic. The problem was inside, not outside. This keyword, *acceptance*, was the opposite of fighting, which was the instinctive response of the panic stricken. Yet it was exactly this fighting against tension, fear, anxiety, and panic that perpetuated the problem.

Weekes' treatment protocol was a simple haiku: *face, accept, float, let time pass*. It was not designed to eradicate all the stresses of life, but to enable people to find their own way out of distress.

'To recover, he must know how to face, accept and go through panic until it no longer matters ...' she told the Fall Conference. 'Recovery is in his own hands, not in drugs, not in avoidance of panic, not in "getting used to" difficult situations, nor in desensitization by suggestion. Permanent recovery lies in the patient's ability to know how to accept the panic until he no longer fears it.'

Weekes work anticipated advances made decades later and her approach has been vindicated. She also changed the way anxiety was understood and treated, yet this achievement is largely unrecognised. In 1977, Zane, who had witnessed the success of her method, even with intractable cases, was dismayed by the reaction of his peers to her speech. 'The thing that I remember was the depth of her observations and the lack of appreciation, it seemed to me, by most of the audience of what she had to say. I, at least, was able to comment publicly that Dr Weekes was a real pioneer in this field and the thing that was remarkable about her was that patients came to me talking about her.'

That was the difference between Weekes and other professionals, Zane says. 'She was coming to us from where the patient is, and not from our top, where we were telling the patient what it's all about, why he is the way he is.'

A few years later, on 7 May 1983, Weekes was back in New York, again a keynote speaker addressing professionals. Again, her sponsor was Zane, who had invited her to make a presentation to the Fourth National Phobia Conference. Again, Weekes explained her approach at length. People could be taught to cure themselves, she said, to find that inner voice 'to support and lead through setbacks, through flash moments of despair, through the bewilderment'.

This time, however, she asked them to look into their void.

'I am aware that many therapists believe there is no permanent cure for nervous illness. When I was on the radio some years ago in New York with a physician and a psychiatrist, the psychiatrist corrected me when I used the word cure and said, "You mean remission don't you Dr Weekes? We never speak of curing nervous illness!" I told her that I had cured far too many nervously ill people to be afraid to use the word.'

It was a provocative claim, but one that sat on an unshakeable foundation.

In the early 1970s, Anne Turner, a young British woman married with a small child, faced the prospect of an operation on her brain, a procedure that she called by its medical name, leucotomy. Known popularly as a lobotomy, it involved cutting into the frontal lobes, with inevitably mixed results.

Turner was 31 years old, from Yorkshire, England. Surgery was now being offered as the last hope of routing her mental demons, the unbearable ruminations and obsessions she neither understood nor controlled. There had been a maze of treatments, analysts, intravenous drugs, hospitalisations, and shock therapy, but the mess in her mind remained. She toyed with suicide.

Stress was not a new experience. Turner had suffered a nervous breakdown at the age of 20 and had electric-shock treatment at the age of 21. She survived these episodes, but, by the time she was in her 30s, with a small daughter, another set of stresses swept her into a breakdown. 'Well, there was a second one,' she says, 'and it got a lot worse, it got a lot worse.'

Terrified of surgery as she knew someone who had undergone an unsuccessful lobotomy, Turner concluded she would rather die than endure the procedure herself. When it was suggested, she thought, 'That's it, I've had enough. I'm going!'

In this state of mind, and quite by chance, she turned on the television to hear a doctor describing her symptoms so exactly that she could have been reading Turner's mind. Moreover, the doctor not only knew how she suffered, and why she suffered, but insisted recovery was possible. Nervous illness, Turner heard, was quite treatable.

At the end of the broadcast, there was mention of a book, and although Turner knew neither author nor title, her local bookshop had no trouble identifying it. 'Oh, that's by Claire Weekes, we've had a lot of enquiries for her book,' Turner was told, and directed to *Self Help for Your Nerves*, which had been published in the UK in 1963, almost a decade earlier. 'Here was a woman writing about me. Everything I had was in this book, and I thought … I can't be so different if someone on the other side of the world can write a book about me. It was a revelation, that book, because it was about me.'

At the back of the book was an address, and Turner wrote to the author asking simply: 'Is there any hope I can ever recover?' She included a stamped envelope and hoped 'with any luck' for a reply. 'By return post, I got a letter back, handwritten, saying, "Yes, there is hope. Here is a telephone number, give me a ring if you want to."'

Turner picked up the phone and reached Weekes, who was staying with her friend Joyce Skene Keating, a local magistrate who lived at Queen's Gate Gardens, London. Skene Keating had contacted Weekes the same way, seeking help for severe agoraphobia, not long after being widowed in the mid-1960s. Weekes stayed in Skene Keating's large, comfortable apartment whenever she was in London.

Recalling that phone conversation over 40 years later, Turner can remember her astonishment when Weekes described what she thought was her own unique experience. 'How do you know how I feel?' Turner asked. She has always remembered Weekes' response: 'I don't have to know anyone, I know the illness very well.'

Weekes explained that the mind and the body could behave as if something was terribly wrong when it was just a reaction to fear. 'I could have been just like you. They are just the thoughts of a very tired mind, and they come back because you are frightened of them.' It could happen to anyone and anyone could be cured. It was 'simple', although not 'easy'.

Turner was buoyed by the personal support this 67-year-old doctor was prepared to offer. Weekes promised to keep in touch, even when she returned to Australia. She would not take payment; Turner could pay for the phone bills.

Turner cancelled the leucotomy. What Weekes said struck her as common sense. As anxiety disorders were not well understood or managed by the medical profession in the '70s, Weekes' advice was better described as uncommon sense. Psychiatry was under siege from within and without, and treatment for anxiety ranged from psychoanalysis, to exposing people to stress while teaching them to relax, to drugs. When all this failed, there was shock treatment.

The overwhelming experience of a panic attack, which could not be controlled or quelled, was not well understood, and even less well treated. The phrase itself had not even been coined. Turner also had what would later be labelled OCD, obsessive-compulsive disorder. Yet here was a medical practitioner who regarded these conditions as quite curable. Sufferers were just bewildered or tricked by what she called nerves. The problem was 'nervous illness'. Weekes' book explained in detail the nervous system and how the mind and body were interconnected.

She was a doctor of medicine, and a scientist, but her approach could not have been further from that of another doctor and scientist, Sigmund Freud. Referring to the legendary psychiatrist's pioneering technique of interrogating his patients while they were prone, Weekes boasted of being 'one of the first to deal a blow at the old Viennese couch technique. I led them out of the consulting room, into the world where they were to live successfully.'

Weekes was heading home to Australia, and she left Turner some tape recordings of her advice. 'Just ten minutes. You don't need long tapes.' They were to be played over and over, to remind the tired suffering brain of the way out of torment.

She would speak to Turner twice a day when she got back to Australia, and for as long as Turner needed. 'I'll get you through the day, and [you can] ring me up at night and tell me how you've been,' she promised. Turner began to recover. It would turn out to be a permanent cure.

Turner was uncomfortable Weekes wouldn't charge her. 'She wouldn't take anything for it. When she went back to Australia, I said you haven't sent me a bill, Dr Weekes, and she said: "No and I never shall. You just spend your money on the telephone calls."'

However, Turner eventually repaid her debt in a different currency. In 1983, when Weekes was a household name in Britain following the success of her books, the BBC invited her to give a series of six television interviews to be broadcast weekly at lunchtime.

They wanted an interview with someone cured by Weekes as an opener for the series, but it was hard to find anyone willing to endure such public exposure. Weekes finally asked Turner, who reluctantly agreed. Telling the story of her breakdown and recovery on television, Turner concluded with the observation that 'if you've not been in hell, you don't know what heaven is. I can truly say that I'm happy.'

Weekes was grateful. She understood the personal cost of a public appearance. 'For Anne to appear on television before millions of compatriots took outstanding courage. She had so much desire to save others from the suffering she had known that she put their suffering before her own comfort. Her story was given so simply, honestly, and intelligently, that she may have helped thousands with it.'

Weekes was making a particular point. It was Turner's story, and her achievement. She always insisted she was teaching people how to cure themselves.

Across the Atlantic, around the same time Turner first encountered Weekes in the 1970s, a small child developed a phobia that engulfed her family. Her father, who happened to be a psychiatrist, found himself unable to help his young daughter. It was frustrating, and distressing. At that stage, Dr Robert DuPont had no knowledge of Weekes or her work.

DuPont had graduated as a psychiatrist from Harvard University in the 1960s. Addiction was his specialty, and he had pioneered methadone treatment in black communities where drugs drove a never-ending cycle of crime and poverty. The success of his programs eventually came to the attention of the US government, and, in 1973, DuPont was appointed White House 'drug czar', in which role he served two presidents, Richard Nixon and Gerald Ford. He established and ran the Narcotics Treatment Administration and was founding director of the National Institute on Drug Abuse.

For DuPont, encountering Dr Claire Weekes was a godsend of timing. He was juggling pressures on two fronts, at home and at work. Not only did he have a child with a phobia, but, with the inauguration of a new president in 1977, DuPont was about to lose his job. 'The Secretary of Health, Education, and Welfare had just come in with the new president, Jimmy Carter, and he wanted to have new people, his people, so I was fired. In 1978, I was out on my ear.'

DuPont turned to full-time psychiatry, where he treated anxiety as well as addiction. There were adjustments to be made, but his most serious challenge was at home.

Years before, when his two daughters, two-year-old Caroline and her four-year-old sister, Elizabeth, were playing hide and seek with their cousins, they accidentally locked themselves in a closet. They were not there for long as the adults soon discovered them, but, while Elizabeth shrugged off the experience, for Caroline it was a disaster. She became terrified of confined spaces.

In first grade, she was confronted at school with a small, windowless bathroom off the classroom. Caroline refused to use it. Elizabeth had to come to the class at lunchtime to stand by the door to give her sister the confidence to enter.

Managing Caroline's phobia involved the whole family. The problems DuPont struggled with in his therapy practice had walked through his front door and yet his professional training offered him no effective tools to manage them. If anything, they invited critical attention to his daughter's early childhood relationships with significant others — especially her parents. Freud's work in psychiatry had inspired the search for the 'why' behind mental dysfunction. Parents could find themselves part of the answer to that question — and not necessarily in an attractive way.

Generations of psychiatrists and psychologists had been reared on Freud. His language — ego, id, superego, transference, repression, penis envy — had only been further complicated by the praxis of his psychoanalytic technique of free association and dream analysis. It would be hard to imagine a more complex yet highly subjective treatment protocol.

In the face of his daughter's ongoing anxiety disorder, DuPont was frustrated. His elder daughter, Elizabeth, who herself became a therapist specialising in the field, captures her father's twin plights: 'Here he had a daughter who was suffering so much, and, at the same time, he had a patient who had panic disorder and had been seeing him for a year and hadn't gotten any better,' she recalls.

One day during treatment, a patient he had been seeing for some years told DuPont about an article she had read in a women's magazine on a new approach to anxiety being taken by the Phobia and Anxiety Clinic at White Plains Hospital in New York. She wanted to try it.

DuPont was unimpressed: 'I'm a Harvard graduate and I don't get my ideas from *Glamour* magazine,' he said. The patient persisted, pressing on him the name and number of the clinic's founder, Dr Manuel Zane. DuPont had an open, inquiring mind and his curiosity was finally piqued. He and his patient headed off to New York together.

When they arrived, DuPont met in Zane another psychiatrist with an open mind. Zane had founded the first phobia clinic in the US, and DuPont was 'just amazed. I saw people with courage confronting anxiety — doing things that had been impossible before. I was totally mesmerised by Manuel Zane, an innovative psychoanalyst who was devoted to his patients and able to help them with their terrible fears.'

However, he found Zane was himself mesmerised by another doctor, an Australian medical practitioner turned self-help writer. So many of Zane's patients had recovered after reading Weekes' books that the clinic had begun recommending them. They had also contacted Weekes in Australia, inviting her to visit.

It was at Zane's clinic that DuPont was introduced to Weekes and her work. He was astonished to see the queues of patients lining up with their dog-eared copies of Weekes' latest book, waiting to thank her for 'saving' their lives.

Reading *Hope and Help for Your Nerves*, as *Self Help for Your Nerves* had been retitled for publication in the US in 1963, DuPont discovered a treatment that was completely different from the prevailing orthodoxy, yet one that 'worked fabulously' with his patients and provided a breakthrough for Caroline. Using the approach of Weekes, his youngest daughter recovered. The experience was a life-changer for the entire DuPont family.

After years of suffering, Caroline, in 1978, at the age of ten, overcame her fear of enclosed spaces. She gave her father a birthday present by riding ten floors in an elevator, alone. DuPont waited below for his daughter as she exited.

'This was a whole new way to look at what was going on with Caroline. Her getting better was a blessing for our whole family,' says Elizabeth DuPont. 'A weight lifted off all of us.'

The experience changed the direction of DuPont's career. He set up the first phobia program in Washington, then established the Phobia Society of America, which later became the Anxiety and Depression Association of America. DuPont believed Weekes shaped history.

'I don't know anyone else I met in my life who has had the kind of impact on millions of people that Claire Weekes had on the big medical and human problems with anxiety,' he says.

Forty years after Bob DuPont and his patient drove to White Plains, one of the foremost contemporary experts in anxiety, Dr David Barlow, professor of psychology and psychiatry at Boston University, agrees that Weekes completely changed the trajectory of treatment of severe anxiety states.

'In the case of the brilliant physician Claire Weekes, her clinical intuition led her to think what was then unthinkable: that someone housebound with severe anxiety and panic ... could overcome these problems by actually exposing oneself to the very situation that brought on the severe anxiety and panic in the context of strong clinical support.'

When Weekes first developed her approach, 'it ran entirely against the prevailing theories', which, according to Barlow, assumed that exposure to a phobia could result in a psychotic episode. 'By thinking outside the box, as we now say, and exercising extraordinary clinical sensitivity with her patients, she became the originator of exposure therapy for agoraphobia to the unending benefit of tens of millions of patients over the years.'

He describes Weekes as a 'deeply experienced and intuitive clinician' who had 'serendipitously' discovered 'important new clinical innovations in the course of actually helping people deal with their disease or disorder'. Yet there was nothing serendipitous about Weekes' 'brilliant' insights. They were hard earned over two years of suffering when Weekes as a young woman had become nervously ill quite unexpectedly.

By the time Weekes met Anne Turner and Robert DuPont, she had a global following of grateful patients and readers. Her understanding of the destructive power of anxiety and panic was the culmination of a lifetime of professional attention. However, it had been her searing experience of 'nerves' as a young woman that had inspired her work. She knew that she could cure others because she had cured herself.

Chapter 1

MISDIAGNOSIS

In 1928, at the age of 25, Claire Weekes was making academic history as the first woman likely to be awarded a Doctor of Science degree at the University of Sydney. With a first-class honours degree in science and the University Medal for zoology, she was aiming for a Rockefeller Fellowship to further her studies in England after completing her PhD. Then suddenly she lost her footing and found herself in freefall.

It started with a sore throat, followed by a botched operation on septic tonsils resulting in a haemorrhage. 'I'd had severely infected tonsils. I'd eaten very little for months and had lost two stone,' she said years later.

For a small, slightly built woman, 13 kilograms was a significant weight loss. In her weakened state, she experienced heart palpitations and was referred to a Sydney specialist she knew as a 'famous cardiologist', who gave her injections of calcium, which had little or no effect.

Fragile, emaciated, and with a racing heart, Weekes was a puzzle to her local doctor, who finally, with scant evidence, made a monumental diagnosis. He concluded she had contracted the dreaded disease of the day, tuberculosis.

'I can remember I thought I was dying,' she recalled in a letter to a friend. 'I was sent away to the country and I was told that for six months I must make no effort, not even to pull a blind down.'

Tuberculosis invoked the terror of the black plague of earlier years and was a preview of the HIV/AIDS epidemic to come generations later. Children and young people were particularly vulnerable to this efficient killer, and there was no antidote. It was responsible for almost 10 per cent of deaths in the early 20th century.

Then there was the treatment. Being highly contagious, TB meant isolation from family and friends, with quarantine in sanatoria strategically placed far from cities and communities. Sufferers were often marked by the illness for life.

For Weekes, the terror of TB would have been quickly followed by the horror of the sentence, a separation from those to whom she was closest. Many sufferers were incarcerated for years.

She later recalled that she had accepted this bad news without question, although there had been no final confirming test. 'It was way back in the 1920s, and I was not X-rayed. Of course, I believed I had TB,' she said later, with exasperation.

Her studies were put on hold, and the young woman who hated being alone was packed off to the Waterfall State Sanatorium, which was located 38 kilometres south of Australia's biggest city, Sydney. At 300 metres above sea level, it fulfilled the requirement for cool, fresh country air.

Here there was no occupation and no one to keep Weekes company in the face of the death and dying around her. Fear touched everyone. Her heart continued to race. 'I was more or less confined to lying on the couch, with nothing much to do, and six months on my hands. So that I knew what it was to become introverted, worried,' she said of that period.

The Waterfall sanatorium was opened in 1909 when the

bacterial disease was the leading killer of Australian women, and very near that for men. When patients were in the active phase of TB, they were isolated in fibro chalets about the size of a garden shed. They either recovered or ended up in the Garrawarra Cemetery, less than a kilometre away.

The long single-storey main building enjoyed a magnificent outlook. Set on the ridge of a plateau, it had a full view of the Southern Pacific Ocean from its traditional wide Australian verandah. For the inhabitants, the panorama must have been a rare solace. Yet however beautiful the view, they had more powerful competition for their attention. There was a death every three to six days between 1909 and 1930, making a tally of about 100 a year.

TB did not always select the underprivileged, but it had a strong affinity with poverty. Claire Weekes did not fit this profile neatly. Her family were not rich, but they were certainly not poor. Isolation and privation were a novelty.

By the time she was diagnosed with TB in her mid-20s, Weekes had already left the preordained path for Australian women, most of whom were destined for domestic duties. Academia was dominated by men in the 1920s — and this was particularly true of science, her career choice, but she was ambitious and hard-working.

Weekes had won a place at Sydney Girls High School, a selective school where she performed with distinction, winning several awards. She matriculated in 1921 with sufficiently high grades to win the Yaralla Scholarship to the Women's College at Sydney University. The scholarship paid £50 annually 'to any student of high attainments who could not afford to reside in college without financial assistance'.[1] She excelled as an undergraduate and beyond. Before she fell ill, she was an academic building an international reputation.

At the sanatorium, there was silence. Weekes was immobilised by her circumstances. In later years, she preferred physical inactivity, but that point was yet to arrive. Now she felt exiled. 'For a healthy young girl, [it was] something to have get used to,' she said with some understatement years later.

She did not get used to it. The sanatorium was the perfect Petri dish for a fear that would grip and not let go. Yet Weekes was one of the lucky ones, for, after six months, the doors of the sanatorium swung open. The doctors concluded a mistake had been made and she had been wrongly diagnosed.

Far from being relieved, Weekes felt immeasurably worse. Now she was convinced that she had a serious heart complaint as the tachycardia — a racing heart — was unceasing. Once outside the sanatorium, she was terrified and overwhelmed.

'I can remember, I had lost all confidence in what I could do, because I'd been told "you mustn't do this, you mustn't do that!" I remember walking out alone and thinking "I wonder if I can walk as far as the corner of that street?" I remember being aware of every footstep I took and wondering how much faith I could still have in my body to get there.'

Rather than immediately returning to university, she chose to recuperate with a female friend in 'the country' who was married to a doctor. Weekes hoped for some advice on her heart problems, but instead she found more medical incompetence.

'I remember … my heart would palpitate if I woke up at night, just the shock of waking up would make it accelerate. I can remember very clearly how, one night, I called out to her when my heart was beating fiercely and thought my last gasp was coming. Her husband, the doctor, said, "No. I won't go to help her. She'll think she's worse than she really is!"'

The doctor, whom Weekes did not identify in interviews when she later publicly spoke of this turning point in her life, was right in one respect. There was nothing wrong with Weekes' heart. She was to live for another 60 years. However, something important had gone unexplained. It was fear that was managing her heartbeat, and, without knowing this, she was trapped in a vicious cycle.

By the time Weekes eventually came to understand the mind–body connection — that her unrelieved fear was firing her nervous system, which in turn fired her heart — she had endured two years of extended suffering, inhabiting a state of permanent anxiety in such distress that she no longer recognised herself. When she eventually learned how to strip fear of its power, she coined a word — 'sensitisation' — to explain the discomfort of exaggerated emotions that followed some stressful events.

Two failures of medicine shaped Weekes' future. First, she had been wrongly diagnosed with TB, a devastating medical error given the consequences, and, second, her friend's husband had left an indelible impression, an example of how *not* to practise medicine. Weekes would eventually go on to become a GP (general practitioner, or primary-care physician) herself.

'When I first became a GP after years of more specialised work, I knew about the symptoms of stress,' she told a popular magazine in 1978. 'I recognised in my patients what I had suffered myself. I had cured myself of stress symptoms after I had a haemorrhage following an operation for septic tonsils. They thought I had TB. I hadn't but there was a loss of confidence.'

She never forgot the doctor who denied her reassurance at that desperate time. 'One word from him then about sensitisation would have saved me two years of worry and suffering but perhaps it was just as well because what I learned then has helped me help hundreds of thousands of people. Perhaps I should thank the doctor.'

After a faltering start marred by misdiagnosis and mental torment, Weekes' misfortunes inspired her life's work on anxiety.

Sitting beneath words destined to be read and understood by distraught individuals and branded as self-help lay a body of scholarship. Yet, for now, her suffering persisted. It would be years before she cracked the anxiety code.

Chapter 2

HER MOTHER'S DAUGHTER

Frances Florence Newland married Ralph Clinton Weekes in the first year of the 20th century, when both were 23 years old. Sixteen months later, on 11 April 1903, Hazel Claire Weekes was born. From the beginning, she was known by her middle name. A handwritten note from an unidentified source, found years later among her belongings, noted crisply: 'CLAIRE BORN Good Friday, Nickname "Bunny"'.

Good was a defining word. Although the Weekeses had three more children, it was the eldest who never disappointed. In 1906, Horace Stanley arrived, and, like his older sister, he dispensed with his first name in favour of 'Brian'. In 1909, Alan Clinton Newland was born, followed a year later by Dulcie Jean.

Paddington, Sydney, was identified on Claire's birth certificate. Far from the expensive inner-city neighbourhood it would become, it was a working man's suburb with long lines of identical terrace houses straggling across the ridge up the hill from Sydney Harbour. It was home to the stonemasons, quarrymen, carpenters, and labourers employed on the nearby Victoria Barracks. The wealthy lived in larger villas down near the water.

The Weekes house at 4 Grove Street, Paddington, was a typical terrace but one of the larger ones, having two storeys. Claire and her brother Brian were born there, but, a few years later, the Weekeses moved further out from the city to Watson's Bay. There was less congestion, the houses were bigger, and beyond the backyard was a paradise of water and land, which offered Brian, in particular, an enchanted childhood beyond the parental gaze. The suburb had a ferry service, a post office, a school, a few churches, and only 100 or so houses. It was perfectly appointed to enjoy Sydney's harbour charms.

Most of Claire's early youth was spent here, and it might have been just another lovely harbourside suburb except for two key claims on history. The little beach had welcomed the first settlers of Australia, who landed there, over 100 years before, on 21 January 1788. When Captain Arthur Phillip arrived with his entourage on the First Fleet to establish the British penal colony, he turned from the ocean into a huge tranquil harbour, stopping overnight at what would become known as Camp Cove, in Watson's Bay, before moving further on.

This historic claim to fame was to be accompanied by a more contemporary, continuing notoriety. The towering headland that separated ocean from harbour was one half of the open gateway into the magnificent Sydney Harbour. Its sheer cliffs, which acted as a great buffer to the ocean, offered a vast view to the horizon. The highest point was known as The Gap. With its promise of an uninterrupted journey in quick time to the rock platform beneath, it became famous for suicides. For instance, when Claire was five years old, a brief note in the local paper recorded that 'George Pinson, aged 18, committed suicide at Watson's Bay today owing to disappointment in a love affair.'

Blue was to be Claire's favourite colour. Duck-egg blue, according to one of her nieces. As an adult, she favoured blue stationery. An ocean has many moods, and blue can be cruel as well as beguiling. At Watson's Bay, residents lived on a rocky, wooded spit of land dividing ocean from harbour, with long views down to where, 30 years later, the famous metal span of Sydney Harbour Bridge would define the city, joining south to north.

The Weekes home at Watson's Bay was bigger than their first and had a garden. It was chosen deliberately by Frances, known always as Fan, who put its spacious ground floor to work by taking in tenants and establishing herself as a co-breadwinner. Ralph was a musician. Fortunately, he was in constant employment, mainly in vaudeville, but also with the Sydney Symphony Orchestra. Still, the extra money came in handy.

Claire's brother Brian would remember their childhood there in the first ten years of the 20th century as an idyll. 'Our Bay had its moments of expectation and the big events, but it was mostly a blue sky, the North Easter, the ferry, the tram terminus, the wharf, the park, the school, the church, shops, swimming baths, lifeboat, Parsley Bay, The Gap, the pub near the park, and the boatshed. The two beaches — the Wharf Beach and Camp Cove. All these places made up the jigsaw of life.'

Life for Brian, the family menace, was the joy of water, rocks, spying on lovers, and tormenting them with tricky torches hung on ropes from trees. Most of the time, he just felt great in his skin. Nothing really like it since. He remembered it all, especially the tenants: 'I was a barefoot six year old knowing full well he had to buzz off before all hell brook loose if he were seen. Watching two people without clothes wriggling and kissing like crazy. Mum made it worse by sending those two lodgers on their way.'

While her young brother was busy escaping attention, Claire was sitting in the spotlight at home. From the beginning, she conformed to her mother's wishes, and Fan was determinedly in charge. More than an equal in her marriage, she ran the show, and the family finances as well. Her husband, Ralph, conceded all ground and referred with respect to what he called 'her business woman's thinking'. She may have been small of stature, but Fan was the immovable family pillar. Strong, tough, and strict, her raucous sense of humour hosted occasional malice. Her descendants remember a dominating, resilient character, one of those 'strong women' they lamented was in decline.

A young lad might find himself offered one of her fruit pies, the ones she had cooked with shoelaces. The sight of the boys trying to gnaw their way through her confection would be turned into a great family story, complete with Fan's gleeful re-enactment of the struggle.

Her father, John Newland, came from a family of builders, and the Weekeses would later be beneficiaries of his property ventures. He was an operator. His business involved demolishing as well as building, and he kept a stash of gunpowder on one of the small islands in Sydney Harbour. Newland also spotted a cunning trade, buying surplus materials from the state government and onselling them to the Commonwealth. 'He made enough money to raise Mum and Dad's eyebrows,' according to her son Brian.

Newland prospered, erecting elegant mansions alongside Sydney's Centennial Park as well as others in suburbs close to the city. He also helped to build Circular Quay, the waterfront welcome to Sydney's business district, and joined the Freemasons, that tantalising secret society of men, with its esoteric rituals and opacity — being neither a charity nor a religion but offering networking potential for the man about town, as long as he was not a Catholic.

The Newlands were successful builders who mainly survived the business cycles, with Claire's great-grandfather William Newland bouncing back from bankruptcy. They built churches and pubs. God and mammon co-existed in this practical, robust family.

Ralph's mob were not so lucky. His father, Philip Weekes, was also in the broader property industry but as an artist and decorator rather than a builder, and was co-partner in the well-respected Palmer and Weekes, established in the middle of the 19th century, under the shingle, *Signwriting, Decorating, Guilders on Glass*. Palmer and Weekes prospered for decades building their reputation for decorative and ecclesiastical art, inventing a clever technique for printing lettering on glass and mirrors that eliminated the shadow on mirrors that spoiled the look of the art.

Newspapers reported on the quality of their work on many of Sydney's most famous projects, including their elaborate glass work in the ill-fated Garden Palace of 1879. This was an architectural triumph, running the length of what is now the Royal Botanic Gardens on lovely Sydney Harbour. It burned down barely three years later, its American Oregon timber going up in smoke in just one morning. It had cost £191,800 to build.

Yet where the Newlands managed to ride the ups and downs of the Sydney property market, Palmer and Weekes, despite the obvious talent of its principals and their decades of experience, had no such luck. In the 1890s, Sydney was in the middle of one of its frenzied property booms. Banks were lending without restraint and it ended badly, taking Palmer and Weekes with it.

On 9 January 1897, *The Sydney Morning Herald* carried a sombre report under the headline 'Suicide of a Sign Writer'.

> Mr Philip John Weekes, of the firm of Palmer and Weekes, well-known sign writers of Elizabeth Street, was found dead by his wife at his residence at Paddington last night. Mrs Weekes and her family saw the deceased at 9 o'clock yesterday morning, and they then went out for the day, leaving him at home. Upon returning at 9 PM, Mrs Weekes found her husband lying dead on the bed. The bedclothes saturated with blood, and a bloodstained

razor was found near. The deceased had opened a vein in his right arm and bled to death. At an inquest today, a verdict of suicide was returned.

Ralph's father was just 50, and the death certificate in 1897 was brief: 'Philip J Weekes: Cause of death, Haemorrhage from a wound in his right arm — self inflicted.' Financial difficulties, a troubled mind, and alcohol were a deadly cocktail.

Many of the Weekeses shared a tough humour, but there was an accompanying frailty. This suicide echoed down the generations, and its first reverberation was on Philip's son Ralph, the youngest of five and only 21 years old when his father died. Ralph assumed the stance of a lifelong teetotaller, but the moods, with or without the drinking, were passed on.

It is possible that Fan's straightening instinct also helped to explain why her musician husband, exposed to Sydney's unrestrained bohemian life, avoided drink. His abstinence, however, was imperfect, and Fan innocently reported to the family how Ralph occasionally missed his stage entries when, in later years, he played percussion for the Sydney Symphony Orchestra. She apparently never made the link with the pub opposite the town hall where he played.

'One night, he mistimed his return and did a very loud drum roll in the middle of a quiet section. She [Fan] said he got into a lot of trouble for that,' his granddaughter Frances Maclaren recalls. She found out, decades later, from the son of a neighbour, that Ralph and his cohorts would 'repair to the pub across the road, after which he would play "most vigorously"'. As Ralph's number-one daughter, Claire, once remarked: everyone has a skeleton locked up somewhere.

Fan and Ralph were married a year after his father's suicide. Several years later, another Weekes family tragedy was showcased in the press when Ralph's sister Amy died slowly and painfully from an illegal abortion. At the turn of the century, this was big news, and every salacious detail about Amy's jailed husband, her lover, and her mother's distress and fury were duly recorded.

Fan had a prickly morality, helped along by her own antecedents. She came from a strong line of Methodists, the most famous of whom, Barbara Ruckle, was a Huguenot, born in 1734 in Ireland, where she married Paul Heck and converted to Methodism. In August 1760, the Hecks emigrated to America, where Barbara became known for being 'uncommonly pious'. Her fierce efforts to keep up the standards of religious observance in their new country earned her the title 'mother of American Methodism'. She was remembered for dramatic flourishes, such as breaking up gambling parties and throwing the playing cards into the fire.

This purifying zeal survived in Fan's father, John Newland, a passionate Methodist and teetotaller who terrorised his grandchildren with threats of hellfire and damnation. 'He could get very difficult about our morals and religious upbringing. It all amounted to me being scared of the devil and burning in hell,' Claire's brother Brian said.

Fan inherited the hellfire, stayed a teetotaller, but dispensed with God in the main. She invoked the Bible occasionally as a parental weapon, but, together with Ralph, she remained unsentimental about religion, the best example being their wedding.

When Methodist Fan and Presbyterian Ralph became engaged, they were under pressure from their respective families to pick the 'right' church, but there was not much agonising done. The young couple decided to choose the first one they next passed, which as it turned out was neither Methodist nor Presbyterian, and so they were married at the St George Church of England in Glenmore Road, Paddington.

Fan ruled the roost, but, when Ralph had his moods, he often took out whatever frustrations he had on his two sons. Neither would forget it, although one would be more forgiving. 'Dad', Brian later wrote in his memoir, 'was a problem. Mum and Dad didn't make us unhappy, but we were dodgy about Dad's temper.' Ralph worked late nights as a musician and had to travel right across the city. Any covert drinking would have added to his load.

Ralph's moods frightened and disturbed his sons. Yet decades later, Brian, who had his own problems to negotiate, expressed some sympathy for a father who came second in their family dynamic. His father was the loser, Brian wrote, and 'fought for his place in the home. Mum was the driving force. It was a pity Dad lost his temper. We gave Mum our attention and took a considerable part of Dad's meaning away from him.'

Fan sat solidly in the centre of family life. She could be fun and was a good storyteller, and there was no better story than a bit of gossip. On this score, Fan set such a high standard that her eldest grandchild observed it was wiser never to be the first to leave the room at a Weekes gathering. 'Our family was very critical of people,' according to Frances Maclaren.

Yet whatever liberties Fan permitted herself, they were balanced by the squad of probities she imposed on her children. Religion back then was an accepted part of everyday life, even if the sectarian wars still raged and their family cared little for strict observance. Fan had severe, puritanical ways, and she ran a tireless moral patrol.

She had seen firsthand what could go wrong when men drank and women had sex. Although she didn't preach for God, she delivered her own sermons on sins, obsessed as she was with temptation. She was on a constant vigil, which began as soon as her children could walk and talk, and was quite happy to storm any personal barrier.

Her granddaughters recall interrogations in their teenage years about sex — Fan could mortify a girl — and her other great obsession was the bowel. Yet Fan had some excuse for this second perpetual preoccupation, as diverticulitis ran in the family, and she herself suffered from it. Reflux was the other companion illness. Few in the Weekes clan escaped some gut disorder.

The women in the family recall Fan with awe, but it was hard being her son. Both Brian and Alan would carry their own specific resentments about their mother, led by her obvious preference for their elder sister. Claire became Fan's life mission, and she afforded this child the respect she denied the others. Her eldest was a model of compliance, and, while Brian rankled for decades over his mother's lack of regard, he eventually conceded she had good reason to 'get behind my big sister'. Claire found school everything Brian didn't. He was the naughty boy, she was the good girl.

Claire was more than just the favourite. Fan discerned an intelligence that drew from her uncharacteristic reverence. Everyone noticed, especially the siblings. 'Claire was a scholar and Mum was her more than proud mother,' said Brian.

Brian hated school and Claire loved it. Education became a passion, captured by one of her lifelong keepsakes: a photo of her first primary-school teacher, Charles Edward Leer, who was killed in action in 1915 on the Gallipoli Peninsula. He was the first of several male scholarly mentors who shaped the education of a woman who would leave not just one but two separate and enduring intellectual legacies.

As her interests and her application were evident at an early age, Claire became the carrier of Fan's ambitions. At the time, gender roles were well defined, but Claire was raised to join the world, and Fan never let her forget that her forebears included high-achieving females — on the Newland side at least.

As evidence that she learned early to think for herself, Claire later recounted the story of the maths teacher who had singled out her answer to a geometry question that differed from his. It was publicly recorded on the blackboard 'because it was equally correct but not a conventional solution to the problem'.

Fan reared her children on stories of her successful Newland antecedents. There was the famous 'mother of Methodism', but more relevantly there was a contemporaneous female champion. Claire's cousin once removed, Dr Violet Plummer from South Australia, was the first woman to practise medicine in Adelaide, in 1897 — six years before Claire's birth. Plummer was a firm advocate for her gender, and her career became a model for her Sydney cousin.

Australia was the second country in the world to give women the vote at a national level, in 1902, the year before Claire was born. New Zealand was the first, in 1893, yet the Australian state of South Australia had its own special claim to female suffrage. Inspired by the example across the Tasman, the state gave women both the vote and the right to stand for state parliament a year later, in 1894. The University of Adelaide, in South Australia, was also early in admitting women to academic courses.

Despite such progressive governance, female equality in the workplace was a long way off. Like many women of her era, Plummer, 30 years older than Claire, battled to practise medicine. The newspapers regularly reported on the obstacles women doctors faced. One report in August 1929 captured the paradox: 'Men who had long been accustomed to seeing women performing the most arduous and trying work of the sick as nurses, suddenly found it amazingly indelicate of them to wish to practice medicine. Dr Plummer was at first hissed at in the streets and enjoyed something like persecution from certain sections of the public.'

One of Plummer's closest friends was the intrepid Dr Phoebe Chapple, another female medical pioneer, who sought to serve as a doctor in World War I only to be rejected by the Australian army on the grounds of gender. With all of the obvious challenges that faced her in 1915, Chapple paid her own way to England, where she enlisted in the Royal Army Medical Corps and became one of a handful of women sent to the front, where her bravery was conspicuous. Amid relentless shelling in the trenches in France, Chapple continued to tend to the wounded.

Her war record called for acknowledgement, but, as women were ineligible for the highest honour for gallantry in war, the Military Cross, a medal had to be invented for Chapple. These were stories woven into the Newland family history. In the 1920s, Plummer joined the precursor to the women's liberation movement — the Women's Non-Party Political Association — which aimed for 'the removal of all social economic and other inequalities which still existed between women and men'. Chapple gave the eulogy following Plummer's death, in July 1962.

Fan and Claire followed Plummer's career closely, and her support for women. A 'Plummer Hall' at the University of Adelaide was dedicated to Claire's cousin, who, knowing of the difficulties female students faced securing accommodation, had persuaded a male friend, Sidney Wilcox, to bequeath his house for that purpose. St Ann's College, for women, was established thanks to Plummer's efforts.

There were skeletons as well as successes in the Newland clan cupboard, but Claire locked the former away and lost the key. To her discomfort, she discovered her great-grandfather William Newland (1807–1883) was a convict, arriving in Australia in 1830, courtesy of the British program of transportation. The convict records described him as '5ft1 in tall, ruddy, freckly [sic] complexion, light brown hair, hazel eyes with tattoos on both arms'.

Along with 192 other prisoners, Newland came to Australia on the prison ship *Royal Admiral*, having been sentenced to seven years jail in the Old Bailey for selling goods stolen from his employer

— prints and books worth 39 shillings. It was an interesting choice of contraband.

The 1970s turned up a second convict directly related to Fan. Not only had Fan's paternal grandfather been a convict, but her maternal great-grandfather James Settree turned out to be the same. Transported for killing a heifer, Settree arrived on the *Fortune* on 11 June 1813. His granddaughter Martha Matilda married Fan's father, John Newland, in 1872 in Sydney.

Claire just blocked the convicts out. Her niece Frances later recalled her aunt's odd reaction to what seemed to the child a thrilling episode of family history. Frances equated convicts to the American Pilgrim Fathers and was hoping for a First Fleeter. She came home from school one day fascinated by a history lesson and asked if the Weekes family had a convict background. 'Oh no, we were free settlers,' her aunt insisted.

After a few years at Watson's Bay, the Weekeses left the house and its ground-floor tenants behind to move closer to the city. Claire was ten years old, and their new home in Adelaide Parade, Woollahra, was a quiet street amid a limited series of pretty Federation houses set aloft a large park.

Fan used the move as a warning to her sons. They were leaving Watson's Bay, she said, so that Brian and Alan could have less of a good time; they needed to be pointed away from the beaches and rocks and the lazy pleasures these offered.

The change of location offered a better schooling opportunity, within reach both physically and academically, for Claire and it had advantages for Ralph as well. His job as a vaudeville musician on the other side of the city had taken an hour and a half of travel for six nights of every week.

The children's early childhood had been a creative period for him. While employed with Harry Rickards' Tivoli orchestra, where he played the violin and the drums, Ralph wrote his own compositions with some artistic success. One of his operettas, a musical comedy called *The Sultana* was apparently played in London, although his family felt he had been 'diddled' out of any money. A gift for words, as well as music, was evident in the Weekes clan — most of the children would learn how to wield the English language effectively and they would profit from it.

Ralph had more than music, however; he was a talented artist whose bush sketches signalled a real visual sensitivity, which he passed on, most particularly to his firstborn son, Brian. 'Dad had a great love for painting big water-colours of boats. Rusty "tramps" being towed by a smokey tug up the harbour — puffy clouds — sparkling blue water. Dad's watercolours were special to me — they grew before my eyes and on wet days had me over a piece of paper sucking my brush,' wrote Brian in his 70s. In his short memoir, he looked back to 'the year, 1911 — the place, Watson's Bay. Sun, blue skies, the beach, wild violets, shivery grass and Camp Cove to fish and swim. Dad, a professional musician, had artist friends who visited us.'

These two moody men, father and son, shared an affinity with art and landscape and although Ralph came second in the home, his legacy of art and music and his creativity was branded unmistakably into the following generations, along with his emotional volatility.

The move to Woollahra meant the children had to leave Vaucluse Public School, and the two boys changed schools a few times before settling into the big public school in Bondi. Claire was sent to the public school in Double Bay, a comfortable suburb nearer Sydney Harbour. By the age of 12, she had her first prize — the 'gold medal for general proficiency'.

Money was an issue for the family, and the education of four children tested the limits of ambition. Secondary-school education was regarded as the prerogative of the well-to-do as there was a cost associated with attending even the public high schools. The private schools were much more expensive, already helping to 'solidify the patterns of class-related difference in employment and living arrangements that developed in Sydney's suburban development from the late nineteenth century'.[1]

Although the Public Instruction Act of 1880 was regarded as innovative, making attendance at school compulsory until the age of 14, the state seemed to turn a blind eye to families who put their children to work, recognising that many working-class families depended on their children's labour. It was not until 1916 that the Truancy Act gave force to the legislation and made attendance effectively compulsory.

Education was valued in the Weekes family, driven by Fan's ambitions for her children. The Weekeses would make an effort to keep their children at school, and were prepared to pay when they had the money. However, they were forced to capitulate to the restive Brian, who left as soon as he could, at the statutory age of 14.

The more biddable Alan, who, like Claire, showed intellectual promise as well as application, was sent to the Scots College, then and now an expensive private school in the leafy, wealthy belt of the eastern suburbs. He didn't stay for long, possibly because of the cost, but at least he finished his schooling, unlike his elder brother, at Cleveland Street Public High School. A few years later, there was enough money to afford to send the youngest, Dulcie, to the inner-city private girls' school SCEGGS Darlinghurst.

Claire, however, imposed no sacrifice. In 1917, at the age of 13 years and 11 months, she was admitted to the selective Sydney Girls High School. Her religion was described as 'EC', her father's occupation was recorded as 'musician', and, in the column for scholarships and bursaries, a 'B' sat against her name, signalling her status as a gifted student requiring financial assistance. Only 400 bursaries were awarded annually by the New South Wales (NSW) state government, and they paid £10 a year for the first four years, after which the amount rose to £20. An annual entitlement to textbooks was also included.

This assistance was welcome as the family seemed determined that at least one of their other children would top up the family finances. When Brian dropped out of school to become a sign-writer like his grandfather before him, he was worried that 'my pay was barely enough to pay my board'. He got 'hell' from his parents when he opened his first pay packet to buy a Sargents pie.

Money was a sensitive issue. Claire remembered in her 80s the guilt she felt having unwittingly embarrassed her father in front of a group of men as he was disembarking at the Watson's Bay wharf on his way home from work. She asked for her pocket money and her father later gave 'her such a lecture for asking him for money in front of other people, when he couldn't very well refuse'.

Sydney Girls High School was originally located on Elizabeth Street in the central business district of Sydney, and this prime location put it under redevelopment pressure. In Claire's penultimate year, Australia's oldest department store, David Jones, bought the site for the then huge sum of £124,000. In 1921, the school moved from the city to the suburbs, closer to her home in Woollahra. This was her final year, and by now she had more than found her place, winning prizes and being elected prefect, no doubt to her mother's great satisfaction. School had an enormous meaning for Claire, and this was captured, along with an inclination for sentimentality, in a short article she wrote about the move from the city for the school magazine *The Chronicle*.

At the time, the school building was regarded as dowdy, although it had historic importance as a courthouse, where the colonists first dropped the historic petition to King George IV for representative government in NSW. The school she would write about with such adolescent yearning had been described as a 'sombre, barrack like building'. Cheerless was another adjective, but Claire was enraptured.

> A brass band in King Street sent regular waves of music across the sea of noises and instead of cheering me, made me sad. For soon I shall witness a death — that of the old school. Never more shall I be able to leave by the stiff iron gate, to cross Castlereagh Street, and to jostle with the crowds until I reach the library. Thence to return once more to the deserted school to collect my books, eat my scone, and set off home feeling at peace with myself and all the world.

'The Death of the Old School' was peppered with youthful self-portent. This was the romantic side she would later pull under control, along with any florid writing. In maturity, Weekes was an especially ruthless self-editor, but her early attempts revealed the young Claire as a 17-year-old with a potent sense of herself.

> Oh, to think that those four walls have encompassed hundreds of girls! That within their area dreams been woven, realised or shattered. That girls have left them to pass down the worn stone steps with disappointment in their hearts, with troubles and cares oppressing them, of which the other girls little dreamt.
> ... But why should I soliloquise thus? You are but inanimate things, mere bricks and mortar, straw and clay and yet it is difficult to think of you as such. For me you will always live, even when unsympathetic hands have reduced you to dust, you and your floors, your desks and your windows. When every vestige of your existence has

flown you and your memories will live engraven on my
brain until the last.

Here, amid the purple prose, was passion, a poetic spirit, and
early indicators of the internal waves, lovely and unlovely, that
would beat against Weekes' mental coastline. Behind the restrained,
capable exterior of a woman who would become a doctor twice
lay an intensity of feeling.

Fifty-six years later, Weekes wrote about the over-sensitisation
of the nervous system, a concept that she would use to explain
the inevitable precondition for anxiety, 'a heightened intensity of
responses': 'Mild anxiety becomes acute; a sad event seems tragic;
a strange sight may be disturbingly eerie; love maybe felt so acutely
that the mere sight of the hand of a loved one moves the sensitised
person to tears; joy may be expressed hysterically.'

Claire finished her last year at the new school closer to home
and in the heart of Sydney's eastern suburbs, where the school
remained. That beating heart kept pace with school demands,
and she showed an early inclination towards piety, although she
was later to be privately but adamantly irreligious. In her last year
of school, she was vice-president of the Christian Union, which
undertook such good works as arranging to take flowers each
Friday to the Sydney Hospital.

She was a joiner, took part in mock trials, was in the debating
team, wrote poems that won awards, studied French, mathematics,
and mechanics, and won the school prize for botany, and even the
Mrs Curlewis Prize for Humorous Verse, a tribute to the earthy
Weekes humour. The word earnest was used to describe her later
academic career, and from her mother she got a strong sense of her
place in the world. Her final school debating assignment was to
speak as the lead in favour of the proposition 'That women should
receive equal pay with men.'

By the end of 1921, she had her Leaving Certificate, with honours in English, botany, and geology and a place in the Faculty of Science at the University of Sydney. Again she managed to secure financial assistance, which allowed her to leave home and move into the Women's College, courtesy of the Yaralla Scholarship. According to the school records, 'along with 12 others, she gained a full Training College scholarship', which meant she would be no financial burden on her family.

Her teachers were remembered with gratitude — a Miss Dunnicliff and Agnes Brewster being named in particular as the 'wonderful women' who taught her at Sydney High. In the old girls' publication, she said she owed her 'love and thanks to the school and her appreciation for the joy in learning and living which they have given me'.

In March 1922, Claire entered the Women's College and commenced her Bachelor of Science degree. The university was still a male bastion. Women scientists were news, and not everybody welcomed the development.

Yet the University of Sydney had an early, robust sponsor of gender equality. On 16 July 1881 the then chancellor Sir William Manning announced 'the full opening of the University to students of your sex. Ladies! And the offer to them, if they will accept it of all of its advantages and privileges and complete equality with men.'[2] The sentiment did not endure long beyond Sir William, nor was it universally applied in any case.

By the time Claire entered Sydney University's Faculty of Science, there had been a history of often active institutional resistance to admitting women to university, the most egregious examples being in medicine. At the beginning of the 20th century, the Dean of Medicine, Professor Thomas Anderson Stuart, was courteous to the women the university required him to admit to his faculty but was, originally, frankly disapproving of the practice. 'I think that the proper place for a woman is in the home, and the proper function for a woman is to be a man's wife, and for women to be the mothers of our future generations,' he declared in opposing the decision of the University Senate in 1881 to admit women as undergraduates.

While he explicitly discouraged women in medicine, it seemed the faculty had a special repellent for those who chose not to heed his advice. Women were failed repeatedly. Then when they graduated, there was a further set of hurdles: how to secure a job.

One notorious case was that of Dr Jessie Aspinall, who, in 1906, was offered a permanent appointment at the Royal Prince Alfred Hospital. As confirmation was regarded as automatic, she was rostered on and had actually worked for ten days when the Conjoint Board of the hospital, usually just a rubber stamper, struck out her name and she was forced to leave. The subsequent furore engulfed the NSW government and involved the state's premier. A local newspaper fanned the popular outrage so successfully that Dr Jessie Aspinall became international news.[3]

It was typical of the times. The first Australian female doctor was educated in the US. Given the barriers facing female doctors, Dr Lucy Gullett and Dr Harriet Biffen had in the early 1920s established the Rachel Forster Hospital, modelled on the Melbourne Women's Hospital as a hospital 'for women, run by women' — Dr Biffen was failed five times (four times in fourth year) before she graduated in 1898.[4]

By the end of 1922, Claire had managed a pass in chemistry, a credit in zoology, and a distinction in botany. She reached beyond the physical sciences, and, in 1923, studied philosophy and a subject called 'Logic and Mental Psychology'.

It was a creditable effort, but, in the first half of her second year, Claire left the Women's College and moved back home, a decision all the more puzzling as she had secured a second Yaralla

Scholarship for that year. The Women's College Roll recorded that she 'left college end of Lent term, May 1923'. She had lasted just over a year away from home. Maybe she missed her family, but it was possible her 'half' scholarship meant her parents had to stump up the rest, and the sacrifice was unaffordable.

Over the years, Sydney Girls High School and the Women's College reported briefly on the achievements of Weekes, her travels and her books, but eventually her profile slipped under the radar. In 2013, over 90 years after her graduation, 51 years after the publication of her first book, and 23 years after her death, the famous selective school celebrated its 130th anniversary. As part of the celebrations, it listed a number of Distinguished Old Girls. Their record on Claire was brief, noting only: 'One of the very early graduates in medicine, specialising in neurology'.

This was right, and wrong. It was true that she studied neurology, yet her life's main achievement went unrecorded. Weekes' global footprint had become invisible.

Chapter 3

THE EVOLUTION OF CLAIRE

If the early education of Weekes was shaped by one idea, it was evolution. Many branches of science were still investigating Charles Darwin's famous theories, and vigorous efforts were made in the late 19th and early 20th century to expand on them and to identify the linkages between animals and humans. In 1924, Weekes narrowed down her academic interest to zoology, which guaranteed immersion in the evolutionary debate.

Her choice of specialty exposed Weekes to one of the finest scholars in the field. A large and generous teacher with a huge portfolio of interests, her head of department was the Challis Professor of Zoology, Launcelot Harrison, whose career had taken him to Cambridge, and who had showcased the utility of his expertise in World War I when he advised the British Army on handling the risks of insect-borne diseases in the Middle East, thus saving countless lives.

Weekes found a teacher who saw women as equals, in life and work. Harrison was a rare academic in this respect, and evidence of his enlightened attitude to women was his wife, the writer Amy Mack. She was his senior by four years, wrote under her maiden name, and was an explicit feminist. This was a mix unusual by the standards of the day, despite the gains of the vigorous suffragette movement.

From 1907 to 1914, Mack edited the 'Women's Page' of *The Sydney Morning Herald*, but also built a national reputation for writing about the Australian Bush, which she referred to in the upper case. Mack's *A Bush Calendar*, published in 1909, was well received and sufficiently erudite to be 'beloved by all natural history students'.[1] Getting to know her well, Weekes saw firsthand how Mack built a career from writing, and the learning that lay behind Mack's popular books and articles.

Harrison was liberal-minded and 'made his department one of the most active and progressive in the University', restructuring courses and encouraging a wide variety of research. His students found this branch of biology 'a dynamic force for the discovery of new knowledge'.[2] In the 1920s, that meant, among other things, evolution. Harrison offered Weekes a broad education into this most contemporary of scientific obsessions, which held the promise of illuminating human behaviour.

Biologists studied living creatures and intensively and extensively described them. Harrison believed this basic brickwork of keen-eyed observation was indispensable as it laid the best foundation for answering the big question: what drove evolution? He came to challenge the idea that Darwin's famous theory of natural selection was the one and only answer. Darwin anticipated the later discovery of genes, a breakthrough itself so dominant it overshadowed other influences that might change an organism, an animal, or a human. In Harrison, Weekes had a teacher ahead of his time, a man who anticipated that there was more to destiny than mutations, or genes.

Australia's creatures held a special mystique. Isolation had shaped the evolution of the fauna and preserved the continent's unique mammals. The marsupial kangaroo and the egg-bearing monotremes, such as echidnas, were locked into older reproductive mechanisms. They were a magnet for international scholars, including Charles Darwin.

Described as an 'excellent and enthusiastic teacher',[3] Harrison was also a great mentor, and many students testified to his support, along with the engine of his enthusiasm.

Harrison and Mack drew the zoology students close, inviting them to their home at Killara, with its beautiful garden on the edge of bushland, for birdwatching. 'Not a flower, not a shrub, not so much as a leaf, nor an insect did he not know,' wrote one. Harrison's gumtree was home to birds he called 'his feathered friends' and he could 'put his hand into their nests and touch them without their minding'.[4]

Weekes was singled out for his attention, and Harrison invited her to collaborate with him on a research project in her last year as an undergraduate. As a result of his sponsorship, Weekes' career milestones mirrored his for several years. She graduated with first-class honours in zoology — just as he had done — in 1925. She won the University Medal for her final graduation year, as he had done. He became a demonstrator in zoology at the University of Sydney after graduation and Weekes did the same. Harrison furthered his education abroad, so did she.

As fine a teacher and scholar as he was, it would be Dr Claire Weekes who would be remembered as a pioneer in zoology, though it would be a career she shrugged off before too long. What she took away, however, was threefold: the importance of observation, the shared inheritance of animals and humans, and how to fit the little picture into a bigger frame.

On the eve of her honours year under his guidance, Weekes was exposed to the great landscape of Harrison's ideas on evolution and how science was best conducted. On a mild spring evening, 19 September 1924, she joined the audience in a large lecture hall at Sydney University's Department of Zoology to hear her professor deliver the first of three public lectures on what he called *The Present Position of the Evolution Problem*.

Harrison, with his international experience, was an Australian unabashed by giants, and challenging orthodoxy was the lesson on offer that night. Although an avowed Darwinist, Harrison argued that natural selection was just one of several credible theories of evolution, and further stirred the pot by declaring his belief in 'the great heresy of Lamarckism', which he defined as 'a belief in the direct effect of environment and even in the ultimate fixation and inheritance of what are commonly called "acquired characteristics"'.[5] To acknowledge the French naturalist Jean-Baptiste Lamarck was to invite a fight. Committed Darwinists rejected his notion that evolution was driven by environmentally induced behavioural changes shaping an organism. Yet Harrison felt no need to declare a winner in the evolution wars, asserting there was 'no single royal road' to evolution.

Supporting Harrison's belief that 'functional adaptation to the environment' was a powerful driver of evolution was his subsidiary argument that it was embryology that offered 'the most striking kind of evidence'. The study of how individual life began from a single egg to develop into a fully formed organism 'shows us clearly that there has been an evolution of reproduction from aquatic to terrestrial modes', he explained.

'As the history of the gradual replacement of the swimming sperm, with its inevitable demand for a fluid environment, by the pollen tube is the most romantic chapter in plant evolution, so the gradual perfecting of the reproductive process to terrestrial conditions constitutes the most fascinating story in that of animals.'[6]

Weekes got the message, and the 21-year-old scholar chose

embryology as the focus for her honours year. Harrison had show-cased the great potential of zoology, how engaged it was with the bigger questions of existence. He was also a modernist, with some traditional reservations. In his final lecture, he identified the 'new experimentalists'. These were scientists attempting to raise biology 'from its pitiable position as a descriptive science to the glorious level of the exact sciences, physics, mathematics and chemistry'.[7]

Harrison welcomed this, seeing the limits to scientific inquiry relying purely on description, known as morphology. 'The trend in zoology is changing. The experimental method, in its infancy, is making rapid strides and its results are so important that they, together with recent advances in physiology, must replace the pure morphology of current textbooks.'

However, Harrison had significant caveats. He never lost his commitment to observation as the foundation for experiment, and was scathing of scientists who called themselves experimentalists but often made wild claims, he asserted, against the observable evidence. This was an implicit warning that uncoupling biology from the natural environment ran the risk of delivering sterile findings applicable only under laboratory conditions. Harrison's view of how science should be conducted was a template for Weekes. 'Between these extremes there is an enormous body of less mercurial workers, steadily accumulating knowledge brick by brick, and experiment is certainly the hope of the future. For the present, however, it need not preclude observation, nor even speculation. Evolution goes on in nature and it is in nature that the problem must be studied just as much as in the laboratory.'

As Weekes began her honours year in zoology, a few words would have been echoing in her mind. Embryology, environment, experimentation — governed by observation in the field, in nature. Her professor had accepted the trend towards experimentation, but he insisted on a training in impeccable viewing of the evidence.

There was no point being a zoologist if you didn't visit the zoo that nature provided. In 1925, Weekes accepted Harrison's invitation to join a small group of scientists on a rugged expedition into unexplored terrain, where she would chase the lizards that gave her a lasting reputation in zoology.

Professor Harrison would steer Weekes to a place in science history. The quality of his early training also set her up for her second career. One of his most important contributions, however, was incidental. Harrison introduced her to a friend of his who would save her from herself and let the first light in to the dark mystery of anxiety.

Chapter 4

MEETING MARCEL

At 250 kilometres north of Sydney, and at a height of up to 1500 metres, the Barrington Tops form a spur of Australia's Great Dividing Range. The Tops are of some geographical interest, being a plateau formed between peaks of ancient granite, dating back 300 to 400 million years. The uplift and volcanic activity that followed about 50 million years ago bequeathed a fascinating, wild topography, and the region is now heritage listed.

Claire Weekes was just 22 years old and had been accepted into the honours stream in zoology when Professor Harrison invited her to join his four-week multidisciplinary scientific expedition to the Barrington Tops, which he said had received little scientific attention.

The expedition was an adventure, as well as an opportunity. In the 1920s, the region was relatively inaccessible, completely wild, and perfectly matched to Harrison's interests.

He was smitten by the landscape. 'The beech forest is one of the loveliest features of this glorious highland, and it wraps in its sombre mystery the innumerable sources of the Barrington waters … you must live with a Barrington stream to know these things. I cannot tell you about them.'[1]

It was January and midsummer, but the weather could be unpredictable at that altitude, and the team would be living in tents. Most of the group of 15 scientists were Weekes' senior in age and experience, although a few other students had been invited to join the group.

As even the basic topography of the of the Tops was then unknown, Harrison's party included geologists and geographers, along with botanists, entomologists, and zoologists. Zoology required some physical stamina when fieldwork was involved, as well as intellectual discipline. Weekes' task was to locate and study tiny pregnant skinks. Australia was well placed for the study of some reptiles, especially lizards. Reptiles held a particular fascination in evolutionary studies because they could give birth to live young, as well as lay eggs.

This evolution from oviparity (egg laying) to viviparity (giving birth to live young) engaged the attention of a young woman some 60 years or more after the publication of Darwin's *The Origin of Species*. Darwin, too, regarded embryology as fundamentally important in tracking evolutionary patterns, and Weekes was in the thick of the scholarly inquisition launched by her mentor.

In one way, she was literally following in one of Darwin's many footsteps. On the voyage of the *Beagle*, he was captivated by Australian reptiles after arriving on the island continent on the last leg of the journey. In Hobart in 1836, Darwin's interest in reptiles almost ended his career before it started. He picked up a snake and was intrigued to find it carrying live young, and that there was no egg. 'The abdomen being burst in catching the animal: a small snake appeared … is this not strange in a Coluber?' he wrote in his zoological diary. In fact, the snake he handled with such scientific interest was not related to the species he identified. It was venomous, a copperhead or tiger snake, either of which would have killed him had he been bitten.[2]

Before she headed off to the Barrington Tops, Weekes had had the wherewithal to pick lizard embryology as the focus for her honours year in zoology. Whether she had selected it herself or been steered towards it by Harrison, it turned out to be a fruitful choice. Lizard reproductive patterns were not well understood, yet held some promise of illuminating evolutionary patterns in reproduction in mammals.

In the light of her later work on anxiety, lizards were a fitting beginning as the 'reptile brain' was a popular, unscientific short-hand for the primal survival mechanism of fight, flight, or freeze, which would become central to Weekes' understanding of anxiety. Every living creature down to the smallest bacteria exhibited this innate impulse. Weekes learned early that much of human behaviour involved the evolution of the autonomic, uncontrolled responses that enhanced the prospects of survival.

A study of reptiles required scrambling around in varying habitats. Barrington Tops was a wilderness, but first Harrison and his team of 15 scientists had to get there. The logistics were complicated in the 1920s. Four Ford cars were required to carry people and provisions into a rugged, isolated mountain range.

'It is one thing to take a party to Barrington Tops, but quite another to get there,' wrote Harrison later. 'Not only did one of the cars go missing, meaning the kit and provisions had to be separated from the travelling party in a borrowed vehicle, but the almost 8-hour trip, which started at 7.30 in the morning, included so many breakdowns on the rutted road to the Tops, that a lot of pushing of vehicles and walking was done.'[3]

Harrison believed the Barrington Tops rivalled the Himalayas in beauty and splendour — 'I do not remember seeing so beautiful or so satisfying a view before'[4] — a reminder of how well travelled he was, like many Australians of that generation. Women were as keen to get abroad as men, indeed they outnumbered their male counterparts between the years of 1870 and 1940, heading to Europe for adventure, romance, education, and serendipity.[5]

A rare gender blindness was evident in Professor Harrison's small expeditionary posse, which included almost equal numbers of men and women. He had invited his resourceful wife, who turned the trip into a friendly competition with her husband as both reported on this scientific endeavour for different newspapers.

Apart from Mack, three undergraduate students, including Weekes, and two women on his departmental staff, Harrison's party included three female science graduates: Dr Josephine Bancroft, who specialised in flies and mosquitoes, Miss Enid Mitchell, whose interest was dragonflies and grasshoppers, and Miss Lesley Hall, who studied geography.[6] Weekes was the youngest and most junior of the team.

The wild beauty of Barrington Tops may have woven a spell of its own, and the length of the expedition — 22 days — would have bonded the team for better or worse. There was plenty of worse, given the rain. As Lesley Hall, who had gone to school with Weekes, reported in an article for their old school journal, *The Chronicle*, 'it rained practically for the three weeks we were there, mostly fine misty rain with great wetting capabilities'.

Harrison and Mack covered this trip in detail. While his entertaining reports were published by *The Newcastle Sun*, which served the city closest to the Barrington Tops, his journalist wife had the bigger marquee in *The Sydney Morning Herald*, with its capital city market.

Harrison's team landed in a waterlogged camp at 3.00 p.m. The camp had not been fully fixed up by their advance party, the tents not erected, and rain, which had been expected to stop, continued all day and all night. Worse was the fact that the kit wagon was delayed. According to Harrison, on the next day, the lucky ones had no clothes as they were awaiting the arrival of their kits, so they could spend their time sleeping 'full fed and warm' for the afternoon. 'The rest draggled about miserably in the long, sodden, grass; nothing short of gum boots being competent to keep out the wet. By nightfall there was scarcely a dry garment in the camp'.[7]

While Harrison predicted double pneumonia, Mack cheerfully reported the local saying that no matter how wet you may get up there, you never catch cold. It apparently worked for her.

It was not until dark that the kit wagon arrived. 'The cheers from the women's quarters were deafening, and it was with difficulty that they were restrained from turning out in dinner gowns to a dreary meal under a tarpaulin, which leaked on to a medley of sodden clothes hung on strings over a smoky fire.' Meanwhile, 'Cooking a dinner, and serving it to scattered tents, with limited appliances, in a driving sleety rain, was no joke.'[8]

The Barrington Tops adventure started as it intended to continue, in the rain. Some of the headings associated with Harrison's five reports gave a flavour of its dampening effect: 'Wet Scientists', 'A Day in the Rain', 'Defying the Rain', 'Illusions Gone'.[9]

At first Harrison and his wife, who were in their 40s, worried about the robustness of some of their charges. This proved unnecessary. 'One or two of the girls, who seemed more fragile than the rest, and who caused us a little anxiety at first, are looking rosier and plumper each day,' reported Mack, who painted a picture of the young women with affection.[10]

The Barrington River was used for washing, and as the young women 'leaned over the stream rinsing their white garments in the clear water they looked like a group of dryads. Fair-haired, dark-haired, tall and short, they were as pretty a group of young creatures as any age or country ever saw,' wrote Mack.[11]

The short, dark-haired figure would have been Weekes, and washing her clothes in the river must have been a double novelty. At home, her mother did the chores, as the family revolved around

Weekes' brilliant career. Fan was a practical woman, but as one of her granddaughters pointed out, none of them ever had to make a bed.

Weekes would have been good company, however, and newspaper reports described her as 'vivacious'.[12] She was quick-witted and loved being around people. One member of the expedition in particular engaged her interest.

The tall, dark geographer, Marcel Aurousseau, was an outsider. He had been reluctantly drawn back to Australia to attend to family problems, leaving his job at the American Geographical Society of New York. Harrison was his 'great friend from university days',[13] and, seeing Aurousseau bored and directionless in Sydney, had invited him to join the Barrington Tops expedition. The newspapers identified him as the leading geographer.

At the age of 86, Aurousseau remembered the trip as a break in an otherwise aimless period. 'I remained in Sydney for the best part of a year. I did not succeed in making myself useful or at any rate earning a living from my own training or abilities, although I did join a small expedition to Barrington Tops led by the late Professor Launcelot Harrison after 12 months of what I could only call idling.'[14]

This was typical Aurousseau deprecation. He was temporarily sidelined, but for family reasons beyond his control. He and Harrison were respected scientists, and both were identified as 'war heroes' although for entirely different reasons — Harrison for saving thousands of lives in the Middle East with his specialist knowledge of insect-borne diseases, and Aurousseau for his bravery on the battlefield.

Yet it was true that Aurousseau jumped from discipline to discipline and country to country and spent years searching for a clear professional direction. The choices were too bountiful. As he later wrote: 'I am a dreamer first ... I have learnt many things, and by some of them have earned a living, although I did not learn them just for that. I could be an anthropologist, a zoologist, navigator, historian, many other things, but they are so intensely interesting that I fear to be involved in them — they would capture me for a while.'[15]

As WWI was not far behind these two men, a few weeks of rain at Barrington Tops was comfortable by comparison. As Mack reported to her Sydney readers: 'Our camp leaders have lived under canvas on active service for years, and there is little they do not know about making a camp comfortable; and with tents well stretched and trenched, with unlimited wood for fires day and night, we have been no more uncomfortable than we would be after a week's rain in Sydney.'

At 34 years old, Aurousseau was 12 years older than Weekes. This was a chance meeting of two very academically gifted individuals. Born in 1891, Aurousseau was, like Weekes, the eldest of four siblings. Both were educated at what would become known as selective schools; Aurousseau attended Sydney Boys High School. Given their age difference, there was no overlap in their time at school and there was a gulf between their life experiences. Weekes had only briefly attended Women's College, returning home after just over a year.

By contrast, Aurousseau had lived on three continents and served in the war after graduating with double honours in chemistry and geology. He received a slew of awards and the University Medal in science, an achievement Weekes would equal the year after they met. This gifted scholar had also served on the Somme, whose battles became a byword for the horror of war. Weekes had not yet been taken hostage by fear; Aurousseau had felt its scorching intimacy.

Starting as a private, Aurousseau, like his friend Harrison, left the army a captain, but not before being wounded 'severely' in the first year of service fighting in the famous, savage battles of Pozières and Mouquet Farm. The official historian Charles Bean wrote three chapters on one four-week battle as Australian troops struggled to push a British line forward just a few hundred metres to capture Mouquet Farm.

> The reader must take for granted many of the conditions — the flayed land, shell-hole bordering shell-hole, corpses of young men lying against the trench walls or in shell-holes; some — except for the dust settling on them — seeming to sleep; others torn in half; others rotting, swollen and discoloured.[16]

Wounded on the Somme in 1916, Aurousseau was sent to hospital in London but rejoined his battalion before the end of the year. There was just one reference on the record of his wartime ordeals in his oral history, given to Hazel de Berg in the 1970s.

The winter of 1915/16, said Aurousseau in his deep deliberate tones, 'was something I hope never to see again. It was *rigour.*' There was a pause before he lightly stressed the last word, but that was that on the horror of war. Many of his recollections inclined to the droll. 'That winter on the Somme, the shell holes were full of water that was frozen so hard there was no liquid water to be found anywhere. We used to send a man out to get a sandbag full of ice!'

On 13 October 1916, King George V awarded Aurousseau the Military Cross for 'conspicuous gallantry', Aurousseau having taken charge of his unit after his company commander had been killed. Back in Australia, the headlines celebrated: 'Honours for Heroes'.

His exploits were unmatched by showmanship. H.N. Southwell, the London Special Correspondent from Sydney's afternoon newspaper *The Evening News* reported in February 1917 that he had been 'invited by an Australian lady to tea at a ladies club in Piccadilly, there to meet a wounded Australian soldier who had been doing things'.[17] That lady happened to be Amy Mack, but her determination to introduce her husband's great friend Marcel Aurousseau, war hero, to the world was foiled. Instead of heroics, the trio talked of Sydney, cathedrals, London, books, music, and 'everything else'. Southwell left without a story.

'I had to try to make Mr Aurousseau tell me something about himself, because he had, on the previous Saturday, paid a visit to Buckingham Palace for the king to pin the Military Cross on his breast, but he is a singularly modest chap, and I got nothing out of him regarding the exploits that won the decoration.' Southwell's subsequent report relied on a few bare facts proffered by Aurousseau, who said he spent seven months in Egypt, 'where he learned a few geological facts about sand, went on to France, and attained his chief experience of war in the dreadful battle of the Somme.' That was it.

The journalist had to lean on the official battle report, which said Aurousseau 'took command when his commander was killed and inspired all ranks by his fine example. During a night attack he led his company forward with great dash till he was severely wounded.'

Not long after meeting Southwell, Aurousseau, who had recovered from his wounds, returned to the front as a captain and, after being wounded a second time, was finally repatriated to Australia in June 1919, having been mentioned in dispatches by Field Marshal Sir Douglas Haig, commander-in-chief of the British Expeditionary Force in France and Belgium. He was also awarded the French Croix de Guerre.[18]

A few years later, at Barrington Tops, Aurousseau found himself drawn to Weekes, who had impressed his friend Harrison with her intelligence and fierce work ethic. They had more than scholarship and science to draw them together. They shared humour and music. Weekes came from a musical family, and Aurousseau, who could play woodwind instruments, ended up with a fine collection of polished wooden pieces, from small to tall, which he told his nephew gave him his understanding of perfect pitch.

While Weekes had verve, Aurousseau was more laid-back. She relished public attention while he had no such inclination. Beautifully spoken, with deep slow tones, he could have passed as English despite a surname that spoke to his Gallic inheritance.

Once the expedition to Barrington Tops was over, Aurousseau returned to Sydney, but, with nothing to do, decided to leave the country. 'It was clear to me I could not do more for my family, I would have to do something for myself.'[19] He did what he knew best, he went abroad, heading for Europe.

It would be four years before he saw Weekes again. When they met next in London, Aurousseau's future would still be unresolved, while Weekes was well up the academic ladder and receiving international acclaim for her contribution to evolutionary scholarship.

Chapter 5

LIZARD BABIES AND THE LIZARD BRAIN

Three wet weeks on the Barrington Tops proved a good investment for Weekes. The adventure laid the early foundations for an international career in science as the pregnant lizards she captured at high altitude, then dissected, described, and mounted, made zoological history.

Harrison was sufficiently impressed with the quality of her work to now invite her to collaborate with him on a venture that formally launched her reptile career. Their joint paper, 'On the Occurrence of Placentation in the Scincid Lizard', was published by the Linnean Society of New South Wales on 25 November 1925. Harrison was the lead author, but Weekes shared the by-line.

One measure of academic success, then and now, was the publication of research, but funding mattered, too. The Linnean Society had been founded in 1874 by Sir William Macleay after he criticised the Royal Society — the earliest colonial institution established to further scientific research — for tolerating publications that were 'not of a scientific character'.[1] In 1905, the society established a fellowship in Sir William's name.

The Macleay Fellowships funded gifted biologists. They paid a comfortable stipend and were progressive, with a clause stating that 'women who are otherwise qualified should be eligible for election to the Linnean Macleay Fellowships'. Weekes, among several other women, would be chosen, helped along by the joint paper on live births in lizards at high altitudes.[2]

Lizards were a perfect subject for embryological studies because, unlike mammals, the evolutionary transition was still on display. There was no way of directly studying reproductive evolution in humans as there were no transitional examples. No human mothers laid eggs. Were lizards able to supply some clues to live birth in mammals?

When Weekes turned to lizards, the contemporary science of the day recognised reptiles — as predecessors to mammals, which gave birth to live young — as being mainly egg bearers. However, Weekes was able to extend the understanding of how and why a number actually gave birth to live young,[3] comparing them with other vertebrates, especially mammals, as they shared similar embryonic or placental membranes. Although these structures were simpler in reptiles, they offered a glimpse into the steps involved in the evolution of mammalian placentation, which first allowed egg-laying on land, and finally live birth.

First Weekes had to collect the lizards, which was time-consuming enough because tiny, *pregnant* specimens were required. Harrison and Weekes secured nine pregnant lizards of their chosen species, noting that many male lizards had died in their efforts, a casualty of the impossibility of telling the sexes apart, 'there being no external difference'.

The work was painstaking. Weekes was investigating various stages of placental development — which started with an egg released from the ovary and ended with an internal food source that fed and supported a baby until its birth. With tiny body lengths of 50–60 millimetres, Weekes needed keen observation and a talent for meticulous dissecting and sectioning of tissues, known as histology. In later years, Weekes credited her scientific training for improving her diagnostic skills as a doctor.

Their paper for the Linnean Society, over 15 pages, referenced earlier international studies in the same field and described their results. While many venomous snakes were known to give birth to live young, only two lizards had been cited as so doing. Harrison and Weekes were able to extend this list considerably, but their wider ambition was to explore how the evolution of the placenta in lizards may have mimicked evolution of live birth in mammals and from there to add to the international market in evolutionary ideas.

'It may seem presumptuous for workers with small experience in embryology to enter the lists against submitted champions, but we feel strongly that consideration from the functional rather than from the morphological viewpoint must lead to a clearer under-standing of the facts of early ontogeny.'[4]

Translated, they were investigating how an organism's environment appeared to be the determining factor in how it adapted and survived. They had a dramatic example to prove their point: their Australian skink, *Lygosoma entrecasteauxii*, showed a startling similarity with another skink, far from Australia, known as *Chalcides*, which had been studied by the Italian scholar Ercole Giacomini in the 1890s.

Despite the fact that these two species were from genera 'not very closely related' to each other, it was remarkable that each bore live young instead of laying eggs. The development of a placenta appeared to have occurred independently in the two species. What they had in common was that they both lived at high altitudes. The environment appeared to be the determining factor in their adaptation. Harrison and Weekes did not hazard an explanation of the means by which adaptation had taken place, but the importance of the environment seemed undeniable.

They claimed these fascinating insights could be applied to the evolution of mammals — that functional adaptation to the environment had been driving evolution. Their 'inevitable conclusion' was 'that placentation is a functional adaptation which, given certain prerequisites, may have risen independently on many occasions before the higher mammals settled down to the placental mode'.

Harrison had been generous in the use of the plural when he talked about *their* work because Weekes' efforts had been restricted to the very observations that provided the foundation bricks from which her theories would later soar. He said as much in a letter endorsing her for a scholarship. However, she followed his example of striving for a big picture explanation of the biological novelties she uncovered as she continued her work on lizards over the next ten years.

After the publication of this first paper, Harrison vacated the field and left lizards to Weekes. He was not only her mentor but became her sponsor. In 1926, Weekes graduated with honours and the University Medal, as well as winning the 'special prize' given by Professor Harrison each year. The newspapers reported that 'Miss Weekes, who is 24 years of age, has had a most brilliant scholastic career', under headlines such as 'Lady Student Wins Medal'[5] and 'First at University'. She was identified as the granddaughter of the late John Newland and a cousin of the Adelaide specialist Dr Violet Plummer. Her father's antecedents did not rate a mention.

In 1927, 15 out of 41 students to graduate with a Bachelor of Science degree from the University of Sydney were women, although the majority of these would be 'absorbed in lucrative jobs in the Department of Education'. In other words, they were to become teachers.[6]

Weekes was planning an academic career. Harrison had singled her out, awarded her his 'special prize', and offered her a job on his staff in the Zoology Department as a demonstrator. She began to study for her doctorate in zoology, supported by a government research scholarship, which entitled her to a room and a laboratory at £150 per annum. This was well below the average yearly wage for adult women in 1928, which was about £250.[7]

It was well augmented by the Macleay Fellowship, which was generous and gender-blind. The average weekly wage for adult women in 1928 was just over 53 per cent of men's at the time. Never inclined to undersell herself, Weekes later used the substantial income she earned from the Linnean Society in an application for another scholarship.

'I was awarded a Macleay Fellowship of the Linnean Society in New South Wales. I retained my rooms and received £400 per annum. I was re-awarded this fellowship in November 1927, and 1928 so that I now hold the fellowship until November 1929. I have earned £950 during the last four years,' she wrote.

Harrison had written personally to the Linnean Society in support of her application for the Macleay Fellowship, making a special note of her gender: 'Miss Hazel Claire Weekes has been known to me for the past five years as a student and research worker in this department. Her scholastic career is fully set out in her application, so that it is unnecessary for me to traverse it. I wish, however, to stress the fact that she is the first woman to whom the University Medal in Zoology has been awarded.'

To ensure this fact could not be misconstrued, Harrison added that 'this award is made with a traditional conservation and indicates a high degree of attainment'. He set out his case at length.

> Miss Weekes commenced research work with me during her Honours year in 1925 and bridged the usually somewhat lengthy gap between student and researcher in remarkably short time. She proved a good technician and

able draughtsman, and soon showed remarkable powers of lucid interpretation in working over sections of the very complicated structures with which she was dealing. In her short paper published with me in the Society's Proceedings for that year, my part was confined to checking her work, and to the expression of the theoretical considerations arising out of it, a side for which she was not at the time competent. During the current year, however, Miss Weekes has worked entirely unaided except for consultation on minor points; has collected her own material, envisaged her own problems, and set about the solution in a way that can justifiably be described as brilliant. She has been fortunate in finding a line of research which promises a very rich field, and which is of far-reaching importance in evolutionary zoology. I venture to suggest that her researches will prove as important on the morphological as those of Dr Murray on the experimental side.

Miss Weekes possesses all those qualities which go to make up an efficient research worker, coupled with an extraordinary degree of enthusiasm for her work. The unpublished results which she has so far obtained make it clear that her line of research is of wide general interest. Her personal character is above reproach, and she has a very pleasant personality and presence.

I have every confidence in recommending strongly the application of Miss Weekes. I can promise that, if elected, she will produce a large volume of work of very considerable importance, which will reflect credit both upon herself and the Society.

The society had a good record of awarding scholarships to women. Although the first ten holders were men, in 1918, Vera

Irwin-Smith, a parasitologist, became the first woman to receive a Macleay Fellowship, and of the next nine new fellows announced between 1918 and Weekes in 1927, six were women.

Weekes lived up to Harrison's expectations. The seven papers she went on to write independently of her mentor made her a seminal figure in this specialist field. She had followed Harrison's dictum on the paramount importance of observation, the indispensable foundation for any new theory. She climbed mountains, collected pregnant lizards, dissected and described them, and used her work to offer an entirely new explanation of reproductive evolution: the impact of a cold climate.

Her reputation was built on these two foundations: her demonstration of three different stages of placental evolution in lizards, and her cold climate theory, itself based on her observations that lizards at high altitudes tended to give birth to live young. Over the next decade, she would build an international reputation from her evolutionary scholarship.

Her early studies directed Weekes' attention to what was shared between animals and humans. She moved on from reptiles, but there was more to her education than reproductive systems. Lizards showed fear, they froze, they ran away, and they fought. Humans did the same.

As a biologist, she observed the nervous system common to all living creatures — those instincts that were beyond conscious control. This was the first brick in understanding the primal brain, which she later understood to be so importantly implicated in human arousal patterns. Weekes had also learned that as organisms adapted to their environment, they changed over time. And this born noticer had been further encouraged by Harrison to study carefully the evidence she saw before her, in life. Evolutionary science could extend from animal instinct to illuminate the workings of the human mind and human behaviour.

Chapter 6

THE SHADOW OF DEATH

By 1928, Weekes was working towards her doctorate. She had the benefit of Harrison's sponsorship, his scholarship, and his example, but then, without any warning, she lost him. On February 20, at the age of just 47, Harrison died of a cerebral haemorrhage. It was a tragedy widely reported.

> Professor Launcelot Harrison, of Sydney died suddenly at Narooma, early on Monday evening. For several days he had been holidaying there and on Monday he was fishing from a launch, when he was overtaken by seizure. Respiratory efforts on the part of several doctors restored normal breathing, but the patient sank and died about 5:30 PM. Professor Harrison, who was only 47 years of age was one of the most distinguished zoological students ever produced by Australia.[1]

The testimonials flowed. Australia had been robbed of 'one of her most brilliant zoological scholars'.[2] 'A gifted and original teacher, he stamped his personality on his students, and Australian zoology has lost one of its greatest men,' declared the Museum Trustees.

Weekes was among those badly affected by his loss. At the age of 25, her ascent had been an uphill climb in good weather. Now she had lost her footing. Professor Harrison's death was the first of two shadows to fall across her path.

While his health had been compromised by the diseases he was exposed to during the war — typhus and malaria — Harrison had been uncomplaining about the serious arthritis he endured, so the man Weekes had known was a strong, vital individual, capable enough of leading a scientific expedition into the wilderness for a three-week period. To lose him so suddenly from a vascular event may have played into some of the fearful sentiments that consumed her not long afterwards when she found her usually robust good health unexpectedly compromised.

The summer Harrison died and Weekes fell ill was, she later wrote to Robert DuPont, very hot and humid. Her 'laboratory was three floors up (no lift)'. Weekes developed a range of disturbing symptoms, including heart palpitations, which 'certainly frightened me and frequently wakened me'.

Two years of suffering were to follow, which began with a doctor's mistaken diagnosis of tuberculosis, condemning her to a sanatorium in the country, isolated from her family, removed from her busy professional life, and with only fear as an engaging companion.

Released after six months, she took a brief, unsuccessful period of recuperation, returning to the university on 14 December 1928, to complete her doctorate. She was by now in a far worse state than when she had left. Barely coping, she felt imprisoned by inexplicable suffering, with no idea how to escape. Expectations were high, not least her own, but there was no longer Professor Harrison to offer support and guidance.

Weekes knew what was now expected of her, and it wasn't resting on her laurels. Studying abroad was a common career path for ambitious Australian academics. Aurousseau and Harrison had left Australia to further their careers, Harrison having chosen Cambridge University in England the year the war broke out, while Aurousseau headed to the United States after the war. Weekes, exposed intimately to their individual histories, followed their example and sought international experience.

From the last decades of the 19th century, there had been a burst of outward-looking energy in Australia as scholars made use of their imperial connections and worldwide networks. London was the magnet as the largest city in the world. For Australians, it was not only the centre of the civilisation, but 'home'. For the ambitious, it offered a launching pad to the world.

'The increasing numbers of Australians — including, and perhaps especially, women — who made the pilgrimage to London over these decades are themselves a symptomatic development of this period of accelerated modernity,' said Angela Woollacott in her book *To Try Her Fortune in London: Australian women, colonialism, and modernity*. 'Starting with a trickle of a couple of thousand per year in the 1870s, the flow of Australians and New Zealanders to England rose to around an annual 10,000 from the late 1880s to beyond the turn-of-the-century and then doubled in the interwar period.'[3]

Weekes was following the template laid down by Harrison to fulfil the last of his E's. She had studied embryology, she understood the environmental influences on evolution, and now she was planning to become an experimentalist. Her path was clear, but what looked like outstanding success had turned into unmitigated suffering. She was now frightened of almost everything — not least of all, failure.

After the shock of losing her mentor, followed by half a year in a sanatorium, Weekes was left with one constant, that rapidly beating heart, often so intrusive it was impossible to ignore. It terrified her.

She had plugged away on her doctorate while concealing her agitation, and presented herself as a confident young scholar with worldly ambitions, but there was a disconnection between what Weekes thought of herself and what others thought of her.

While her heart battered away unsettlingly inside her chest, the pressure mounted. Harrison, widely known in London in scientific circles given his wartime experience, as well as his stint at Cambridge, had seen to it that her fresh insights into reproductive evolution in lizards were on the international radar. He had drawn Weekes' lizard research to the attention of Professor William MacBride, a well-known British zoologist from the Imperial College of Science and Technology.

This was especially useful given Weekes intended to apply for a Rockefeller Fellowship to support a two-year research placement at University College London. MacBride was willing to provide references for her to the Rockefeller Foundation. He noted that he had 'never met Miss Weekes, but I have been greatly interested in the work begun by the late Professor Harrison, and continued by Miss Weekes, on the development of a placenta in many species of viviparous lizards'.[4]

MacBride was an eminent, albeit controversial, zoologist, who favoured Lamarck over Darwin in the ongoing evolution wars and was highly quarrelsome, so although it was an asset to be internationally recognised, it was not an unalloyed blessing. MacBride was also a eugenicist who had suggested there was a case for 'sterilising by vasectomy' any man who earned under £400 a year.[5] Weekes, as a woman earning more than that, jumped that hurdle!

Regardless of his views on social engineering, MacBride believed Weekes' work filled in some of the gaps in the picture of reproductive evolution. 'That an organ should be independently developed, not once, but several times, which mimics the well-known placenta of the higher animals, is an extraordinary phenomenon which seems to me to throw much light on variation and evolution,' he wrote, concluding that 'it would be in the interest of science that Miss Weekes should be enabled to continue this investigation'.

Although not in the best state to be making career-defining decisions, Weekes' plan was nonetheless ambitious. She aimed, as an experimentalist, to link her lizard work to help explain the evolution of the placenta in marsupials and mammals. It was out of the field and into the laboratory.

The University College London's Department of Anatomy suited her for several reasons. To begin with, it was home to an Australian scholarly cabal of standing in her field. Furthermore, Weekes would not be the first female Australian scientist to study there, the path having been broken in 1924 by another zoologist, Dr Gwyneth Buchanan from the University of Melbourne.

More pertinently, under the chair of embryology, Professor James Hill, she would be working with a man known as a 'master' in her field. The Scotsman's career had been launched in Australia decades earlier, where, like Weekes, he had been a demonstrator in the Department of Zoology at the University of Sydney. Hill had been drawn to the local fauna that so seduced scholars searching for missing links in the evolutionary sequence, the marsupials and monotremes — the latter, such as the platypus and the echidna, being egg layers — which provided possible clues to the transition to live birth in mammals.

The most important Australian connection, however, would be the head of UCL's Department of Anatomy, the intellectual omnivore Sir Grafton Elliot Smith. Neuroanatomy was his main field of expertise, and evolution of the primate brain was his specialty, among his huge portfolio of academic interests. Internationally renowned, Elliot Smith was one of the most famous and controversial scientists of his generation. He leapt disciplines in a single bound, much to occasional chagrin and argument among some of his colleagues. In this respect, UCL, which was contemporaneously described as 'the home of rebels and agnostics', suited him perfectly.[6]

Hill knew of Weekes' work, Elliot Smith of her reputation, and both men remembered the late Launcelot Harrison well. The three shared career highlights, having all won the Haswell Prize for zoology at the University of Sydney.

Once Weekes settled on UCL, she needed to secure funding support — and had timing on her side. The Rockefeller Foundation had recently provided a new pot of money to fund Australian research.

Established in 1913, the foundation was one of the first, largest, and most important philanthropic money trees, built as it was on the wealth of the Rockefeller's Standard Oil, with the official objective of 'promoting the well-being of humanity throughout the world'. The family philanthropy inevitably attracted local critics, who talked of their 'pervasive influence' as early as 1917, when James McKeen Cattell, the editor of *Science*, complained they had 'undertaken to dictate educational affairs all over the country and all the way from the primary school to the University'.[7]

By the end of World War I, science had become a handmaiden to American power. Scientific institutions were increasingly coming to rely on the generosity of the Rockefeller Foundation, an unofficial arm of soft diplomacy, in preference to government, and thus began a 'steady and close cooperation between academic science and the private sector'.[8]

As America flexed its global muscles, Australia was on the foundation's radar, and the money was welcome as the Australian research funding base was embryonic. Weekes was in the right field at the right time as the natural sciences, social sciences, medicine, and public health were the main beneficiaries of Rockefeller grant monies.

Elliot Smith had good connections in the Rockefeller Foundation having been the intermediary between the foundation and the University of Sydney. He was an important supporter for Weekes given his indefatigable networking skills. His former students made up a worldwide academic diaspora running university departments around the globe.

Weekes easily rounded up referees for her application for a Rockefeller Fellowship. Even Harrison provided a posthumous word with a few sentences lifted from his original endorsement for her Macleay Fellowship. Professor William Dakin, Harrison's successor in the Chair of Zoology, described Weekes as a 'brilliant success in a special field', adding she had demonstrated her 'originality'. He also did a bit of useful name-dropping, noting that he 'happened to be in London last year when her research work was discussed and praised very highly by Professor MacBride'.[9]

His colleague Professor Patrick Murray — with whose work Harrison had once favourably compared Weekes' — wrote he had 'formed the highest opinion of her capabilities and earnestness. Miss Weekes combines very high intellectual equipment with a habit of very hard work and has in consequence been decidedly successful in her investigations. She is undoubtedly one of the best investigators this department has had the honour to train, and I do not think there is any doubt that she will more than justify herself if awarded a scholarship.'

Murray did not forget to speak on behalf of Weekes' most important, but now silenced, advocate. 'I sincerely hope that her application will be successful, and I may also say that, had he been still alive, the late Professor Launcelot Harrison would certainly have been anxious to lend his help by contributing a supporting letter, for he shared with all who knew her a lively appreciation of

Miss Weekes' high abilities and talents.'

The Linnean Society swung in behind her with the secretary, Arthur B. Walkom, declaring that 'the Society has had every reason to be satisfied with her appointment, for she has continued her researches on placentation in various snakes and lizards and has achieved interesting and important results which have a bearing on the subject of placentation in the Mammalia in general.

> From my personal observation of her work I have no hesitation in affirming that she has not only the capacity for carrying on this work, but she has also that rare enthusiasm for her work which is so necessary for successful research. I am of the opinion that her appointment to a Travelling Fellowship would produce results most satisfactory to the Board making the appointment and I strongly support her application.

Weekes' personal application included her academic record and listed her prizes: the Haswell Prize for zoology, Professor Harrison's prize for zoology, the Caird Scholarship, the University Medal, and the Government Research Scholarship.

> I have completed four years of research work. During 1925 I studied the placentation of reptiles under the guidance of Professor Harrison. During 1926 I continued research work on reptiles and collected my own material, which necessitated travelling many thousands of miles into sometimes trackless country.
>
> I was in this way able to supply research workers at the Medical School with material. [Zoology was often linked to medical schools in that era.] During 1927 and 1928 I wrote three papers, in one of which placentation

in snakes is recorded for the first time.

She claimed her work had evolutionary significance beyond the lizard and pointed out it had international recognition.

> During the current year I discovered an interesting condition of placentation in the lizard which, I hope, will enable me to throw some light on the evolutionary significance of the placenta in marsupials and other mammals. This work is considered to be of importance by Professor MacBride from whom I am the honoured recipient of a letter of congratulations.

Her ambition was to do experimental work, and she needed overseas experience as she had 'covered Eastern Australia so thoroughly that I practically exhausted the supply of material necessary for my research work, so the work I have undertaken necessitates a thorough study of all viviparous reptiles'.

Then she made her bold pitch. 'I hope to eventually publish a detailed account of the placentation of reptiles and of its bearing on the placentation of the Mammalia. This will necessitate experimental as well as morphological work. However, I wish to stress the point that I would not be travelling merely as a collector of material.'

In other words she was no mere morphologist, or describer, but was a thoroughly modern scientist. She had some 'interesting problems in experimental embryology envisioned which have gained the approbation of experimentalists in Sydney'. She hoped to work with Professor Hill, and applied for a two-year scholarship, adding that she would like to start immediately. There is no record of what experimental study she had planned.

On completion of her research, Weekes planned to return to

Sydney, where she would either take up her old job as a lecturer in zoology at the University of Sydney, or as a lecturer in anatomy at the Medical School at the same university. 'The latter position has already been offered to me.'

With this weight behind her, Weekes won the generous fellowship, but only for one year. The process had taken six months. On 28 June 1929, W.E. Tisdale from the Rockefeller Foundation wrote to offer it to her for 'a period of not more than 12 months, for the academic year 1929/30, beginning about October 1, 1929, with a stipend at the rate of $120 per month for living expenses, together with the necessary fees for tuition and equipment, if any, and travel expenses from Sydney, Australia to London, England and return, to enable her to study placentation of reptiles at the University of London, with Professor JP Hill.'

Weekes had already completed her thesis and within a year she would be awarded her Doctor of Science degree. Such was the quality of her work that a zoologist at the Australian Museum, James R. Kinghorn, in his scholarly paper on a new species of *Lygosoma* from New South Wales, announced that he had 'named the species *Lygosoma weekesae*, after its discoverer, Dr Claire Weekes, BSC'.[10] On the surface, she was an unqualified success.

Chapter 7

SINKING AND FLOATING

On 22 August 1929, an unsteady Weekes boarded a Dutch liner for a sea voyage to London that took well over a month. The SS *Nieuw Zealand* and its sister vessel the SS *Nieuw Holland* were regarded as two of the most graceful prewar liners to operate between Australia and Asia. At 26 years of age, Weekes had a professional record that eluded most men of her generation. She headed abroad with honours, a doctorate, a scholarship, and the backing of eminent scientists in her field.

The long trip to Europe offered the fascination of brief stops at ports in Asia, yet, as she started on the journey, all she could think about was her racing heart. 'In 1929 I sailed from Sydney to England, to the University of London, still with palpitations!' she reported later. She was certainly excited, but the distractions were internal and infernal.

Fortunately, given her aversion to solitude, she was accompanied by a friend, Cecily Vance. The Women's College reported on their departure for London in its magazine of 4 August 1929, noting that Weekes 'proposes to work at the London University [sic]'. Vance was mentioned in passing as a 'keen student of architecture'.

The two women had met at Women's College. An arts grad-uate and a year older than Weekes, Vance came from a prosperous and successful business family. Her enterprising father, having started employed life as a storekeeper in the small regional town of Kiama went on to build significant wealth as a partner in Clyde Engineering, which profited from the rolling wave of industrialisa-tion at the end of the 19th century. He had died just a year before Vance set out for London with Weekes.

Unlike Weekes, for whom a scholarship to attend the Women's College was more than useful, Vance — known to the Weekes clan as Suze rather than Cecily — came from a family who had no trouble paying the bill. The relationship that was formed between these two young women would last a lifetime and hold a special meaning for Weekes.

Given their proximity at sea, Vance saw Weekes at her most vulnerable, distressed as she was by her rogue heartbeat and its companion, fear. Unexpectedly, nature came to the rescue. The movement of the ocean helped camouflage the palpitations, and soon the voyage not only offered relief but buoyed Weekes with hope that she had permanently recovered from her unknown affliction. She regained her composure and, for the first time in almost two years, began to feel more like herself.

'The journey by ship was wonderful because the rhythm and vibrations of the ship saved me from noticing the vibrations of my body,' she told a reporter when she was in her 80s. The remission afforded her by the rocking cradle of the sea also revived her natural extraversion, and she was one of the more popular passengers on the boat. Over 50 years later another passenger on the *Nieuw Zealand* remembered her distinctly. She said Weekes had a personal magnetism and was always surrounded by people, as she had 'quite an aura about her'.[1] She and Weekes built a good friend-ship on board, and stayed in contact after they arrived in London, eventually climbing the Pyrenees together.

Weekes liked people and did not shirk intimacy, and, because she invested in them, she always had a travelling companion when abroad in later years, as well as a home to go to. She was never short of invitations to stay with someone and had no hesitation in accepting them.

On board and newly vital, she befriended a number of individuals, including a married couple: Tettje Clasina Clay-Jolles, one of the first women scientists in the Netherlands, and her husband, Jacob Clay. They had been posted to Java, where Clay was Professor of Physics at the Institute of Technology in Bandung, and they were returning so that he could take up a posting as a professor of experimental physics at the University of Amsterdam. The pair were renowned for a collaboration that led to a discovery that atmospheric radiation varied according to geographic latitude, which was hotly contested at the time but ultimately proved correct.

Weekes also linked up with a Dutch girl, Dieneke Merz, who had boarded the *Nieuw Zealand* in Java, and, in later months, they biked together around the Netherlands. Dieneke would become a friend for life. Meanwhile, the sea journey consolidated the friendship with Vance.

Weekes' arrival in London coincided exactly with the end of the roaring '20s. On Tuesday 29 October 1929, Wall Street crashed, ushering in the Great Depression. The financial world was in a funk that would last for years. Fear was the motif of the times.

Onshore, Weekes was reclaimed by her beating heart. 'When I arrived in London the sudden quietness after being on board a ship meant that I was once more listening to my own body. I was afraid of my own reactions, frightened by them, worried by them, so I didn't want to be alone in the quietness. I wanted to be always with people.'

She was back to the same old pattern. At night, she would just be dropping off to sleep when she woke with a start. Her heart would be racing, which quickly led to palpitations. 'Then I would sit up for hours for fear that I would die if I lay down.'[2]

The return of her symptoms was devastating. Now there was no way out. The potency of this experience would inform her advice, many years later, to patients and readers. She knew the return of fear carried with it real despair, the death of the hope so badly needed but impossible to secure.

In the self-help books on anxiety that she would write in her late 50s, Weekes had a typically practical word to describe this state: simply, a 'setback'. It was not defeat, she counselled, but was instead to be embraced as an opportunity to practise. Stress, fear, and panic could return, but it was possible to learn how to ride the terrifying waves back to the shoreline. In this way, what she would later call 'the habit of fear' could be broken.

For now, however, Weekes was a young researcher in London. Although she never wrote her personal story, a few words in her fourth book surely described the 26-year-old woman standing in terror on London soil in 1929. When fear returned, Weekes wrote, an anxious inner voice had a 'heyday. It says, "it's all back again! Every lock, stock, and barrel. Every member of the family! We're all here. What are you going to do now? You will never recover now, you know!"'[3]

She felt keenly the paradox of her situation: 'I had everything to live for and I knew it, I had achieved so much, the whole of life lay before me, but I was incapacitated.' Weekes had just arrived in London and yet felt close to collapse. Not long after she began working in her lab at the UCL a friend came 'flying up the stairs' to meet her. She was beyond dissembling, and her first words to him were: 'Oh John I can't take this any longer. I've had it!'[4]

When told of her racing heart and indescribable distress, far from being surprised or concerned, he shrugged. 'That is nothing,' he said. 'Those are only the symptoms of nerves. We all had those in the trenches.'

He told Weekes that her heart continued to race because she was frightened of it. It was programmed by her fear. This made immediate sense. 'All the time I have been doing this to myself?' she asked. 'He said "yes" and laughed,' she later recounted.

His words spoke to the scientist in Weekes. War offered empirical examples: soldiers got scared, their hearts raced, and often continued to race after the threat had passed. John had noticed they then became distressed by their racing hearts, which further aroused and primed them for panic. Yet there was nothing wrong with their hearts. They were consumed with a fear that *felt* overwhelming in the body and so the mind concluded something was terribly wrong and continued to feed the fear.

Weekes had experienced the tenacious loop between mind and body, and here it was explained by someone all too familiar with it: a soldier. Of all the emotions, the feeling of fear was primal. This was the instinct for survival. Once frightened by the feelings in her body, Weekes had kicked off a vicious cycle.

She had already discovered that fear could not be extinguished by the rational brain. Thinking inevitably lost the battle to *feeling*. Weekes' substantial cognitive abilities, which delivered scholarships, awards, and opportunities, were sidelined by an all-consuming dread. It was this *feeling* she was desperate to extinguish, this *feeling* against which she fought so futilely, this *feeling* that was accompanied by racing panicked thoughts.

The discovery that she had been frightened of fear itself was a profound revelation. Weekes was shocked that not one of the handful of doctors and specialists she had consulted had explained how fear could have such a deranging effect on the body.

She immediately grasped the point that she needed to stop

fighting the fear, which was an instinctive response yet counter-productive. There was no benefit gained by striving, trying to think rationally, or attempting to exercise willpower. She later reported it as the breakthrough insight.

'After my friend told me the cause, I just lay as calmly as I could, "OK, I'll just go to sleep, palpitating if necessary."' Once she ceased engaging so intensely with her symptoms, her heartbeat returned to normal. 'The whole thing cleared up,' as she put it. Once she understood 'fear' was bluffing her, she decided to ignore the messenger. She accepted the palpitations instead of fighting them. No battle, no fighting. The keyword was acceptance.

The turnaround was swift. If Weekes had been devastated by her lack of understanding of what ailed her, she now felt exhil-arated, liberated by an explanation from what had been incom-prehensible suffering. With this new understanding, she regained control.

Within a month of John's helpful words, Weekes believed she was cured and was soon 'climbing mountains in Switzerland'. But it was not quite as simple as she presented it years later. The man was not 'John' but Marcel Aurousseau, his distinctive name and reputation camouflaged for a public audience. Moreover, this blinding insight did not augur the end of her anxiety for a lifetime but instead ushered in understanding and a steady path forward.

The thread that ran through her developing understanding of fear was biology. However, the frightful experiment of WWI, of which Aurousseau reminded her, was just as relevant. War's labo-ratory tested minds as well as bodies, with effects on the nervous system that had relevance for peacetime. Science had not taught the soldier Aurousseau that while he must fight a war, he must disarm in the face of fear beyond the battlefield — how he learned this, Weekes did not say. Yet it worked for him, and then it worked for her.

Aurousseau had planted the seed for the bestselling books that Weekes would eventually write, but years of professional medical experience were needed to shape this single brilliant insight of acceptance into a comprehensive understanding of the anxiety state. Meanwhile, the youthful Weekes still had a lot to learn about her own patterns of anxious arousal.

In her books, Weekes identified what she called 'the simpler form of nervous illness', which was what she had endured. Life and further medical education would teach her about more complicated states. Still, it was exactly the simplicity of Aurousseau's explanation that struck her with such force. 'One simple explanation had cured me on the spot!' she wrote. 'Can you wonder why I always go for simple explanations now? You see, I had never gone to bed with "nerves"; in fact, I had fought too vigorously.' In the margin of her typed letter, she added in her tiny tight handwriting: 'Hence my "don't fight."'[5]

The other revelation was that her suffering had been so long and the cure so swift. Two years of mental torment were almost instantly relieved by a credible explanation. Not every reader of her books would find recovery as instantaneous, but, like her, many were relieved to be given an understanding of their bewildering and terrifying state.

In her first book, Weekes camouflaged her personal story by telling it in the third person. A 'student' who had a 'banging heart, sweating hands and churning stomach' and who had done all they could to 'fight it'. A 'friend' who explained that many soldiers at the front had nerves like this, until they realised they were only being bluffed by them. 'He advised the youth to stop being bluffed by his nerves, to float past all suggestion of self-pity and fear and go on with his work.'

If acceptance was the destination, floating was the carriage. It was yielding, the very opposite of the reflexive response of body and mind. You let go, you relinquished will. You 'floated'. This was art as well as science. The concept of 'floating' was redolent of Zen Buddhism rather than Western empiricism, and the seed planted by Aurousseau became fundamental to Weekes' later treatment plan. Of all her simple concepts, it was the hardest to explain, yet was an important component of the acceptance she advocated.

It was easy to confuse 'floating' with 'relaxing', but they were quite different. 'It is certainly relaxing,' she later wrote in her fourth book, 'but it is more than that; it is relaxing with action. One faces, relaxes and then floats on through. Floating does not mean lying and gazing at the ceiling and thinking, "I don't have to make any effort, give up the struggle. I'll just lie here on the bed forever and do nothing!"'[6]

Aurousseau had also briskly advised getting on with work and shedding the self-pity. This invoked stoicism, with its implicit value system, yet it was practical advice that worked. A person occupied — 'floating forward into action', as Weekes later wrote — was more likely to break the habit of hitting the alarm button, than an inert, distressed figure attempting to relax on a bed.

> The sufferer practising letting his body float up from his fatigue has no need to search for a way to recovery. It is as if he steps aside from his body and lets it find its own way out of the maze. The body that so skilfully heals the physical wound without our direction can also heal sensitised nerves if given a chance and not hindered by inquisitive fingers picking at the scar. Float, don't pick.[7]

Chapter 8

DARWIN AND THE HEART
OF THE MATTER

'I was also troubled with palpitations and pain around the heart, and like many a young man, especially one with a smattering of medical knowledge, was convinced that I had heart disease.'

CHARLES DARWIN[1]

Charles Darwin knew all about a rapidly beating heart and the frustration of being unable to control it. Fear could take a man hostage. Sensitive and intelligent, Darwin suffered lifelong bouts of illness as well as anxiety. Yet rather than inhibit his scholarship, anxiety shaped the direction of his interest. Much is known about the famed Second Voyage of the *Beagle* and its relationship to Darwin's seminal works, but the trip was also memorable for the uncharted and uncontrolled internal waters that roiled him.

Even when he set out, at the age of 22, Darwin experienced bouts of tachycardia. By the time the intrepid scientist returned, one scholar described him as an 'invalid',[2] another as an 'invalid recluse',[3] while still another claimed Darwin was 'ill almost continually' for the entire five years that he was on the HMS *Beagle* trip.[4]

Those early expeditions remain remarkable from a modern perspective. For those of nervous disposition, the maritime hydrographic missions of the 19th century and the early part of the 20th were not conducive to relaxation. They were long and arduous, marrying terrifying seas and barren isolation for years on end. If Darwin had looked to history as a guide, then the precedent of the First Voyage of the *Beagle* would not have reassured him.

On this maiden journey, Captain Robert FitzRoy, an English officer of the Royal Navy and a scientist whose specialty was meteorology, was to find himself unexpectedly thrust into the command of the voyage after Captain Pringle Stokes shot himself when travelling through the miserable churning waters off Tierra del Fuego in August 1828.

FitzRoy was later appointed commander of the Second Voyage. By this time, he knew that when things got bad at sea, men could go mad. There had also been a suicide in his own family. His uncle Viscount Castlereagh had cut his own throat in 1822 while in government office.

Planning his second command of the *Beagle*, FitzRoy prepared not only for the tempests without, but for those within. He needed a human investment in his sanity, and protocol forbade befriending anyone of lower rank. Darwin, a social equal, was chosen for this character-building journey by a captain as much in search of psychological security as scientific credibility.

Darwin may not have appreciated his designation as a sanity saviour, yet he understood when he joined the expedition that his scientific interests ran second to the main mission of the *Beagle*, which was to map the permanent temperament and passing moods of the oceans to help ensure safe passage for future sailors.

Whatever its maritime achievements, the Second Voyage of HMS *Beagle* shaped the history of science. Darwin's naturalist studies on this voyage underpinned *The Origin of Species*, published in 1859. It was followed by *The Descent of Man* in 1871. Here was another tribute to the scientific value of an attentive eye as well as an attentive brain. Meticulous attention to detail formed the basis of Darwin's theory and gave it authority. Despite being afflicted by a combination of ill health and nervous energy, Darwin achieved a prodigious body of work. He diagnosed his own problem as over-arousal. There was no talk of problems with his thoughts, it was all about his emotions, his uncontrollable emotional response. Such was his sensitivity that even joy was a challenge.

'I suffer severely from ill health of a very peculiar kind, which prevents me from all mental excitement, which is always followed by spasmodic sickness, and I do not think I could stand a conversation with you, which to me would be so full of enjoyment,' he wrote to a friend in 1862.[5]

Even enjoyment, in the overly sensitised individual, could be felt over-keenly, as Claire Weekes herself later noted. Darwin would have known that the other side of the coin was bleaker still — that stressful experiences were even more fully amplified. Thus his defence was to avoid anything that might give his nerves a workout. Far from accepting his symptoms, Darwin withdrew, a pattern repeated over and over by the nervously ill, and one that Weekes would later seek to break.

Yet he proved what Weekes learned for herself, that even with his well-chronicled ill health, much could be achieved, and Darwin's name was to be synonymous with the theory that would shape science for generations. This possibly explained why his first two books eclipsed his last, *The Expression of the Emotions in Man and Animals*.

This pioneering study,[6] written in 1872, extended Darwin's scholarship into the barely charted oceans of the mind, which so intrigued and disturbed him. It earned him the moniker of 'the first psychologist', yet it was written from an evolutionary, biological perspective. Darwin identified separate emotions, such as anger, fear, and disgust, and his detailed study of facial expressions led to his conclusion that there were universal expressions of emotions, which were found in other species as well and had evolutionary significance.[7] Emotions for Darwin had a functional purpose, and their bodily expressions were driven by biology and evolution.

'With mankind some expressions, such as the bristling of the hair under the influence of extreme terror, or the uncovering of the teeth under that of furious rage, can hardly be understood, except on the belief that man once existed in a much lower and animal-like condition,' Darwin wrote.[8]

He extended his evolutionary theory to emotions by applying his understanding of inherited behaviours — innate animal responses. Although he allowed for some possibility of inheriting learned emotional behaviours, his fundamental point was that the *expression* of some strong emotions could not be controlled.

> That the chief expressive actions, exhibited by man and by the lower animals, are now innate or inherited — that is, have not been learnt by the individual — is admitted by every one. So little has learning or imitation to do with several of them that they are from the earliest days and throughout life quite beyond our control; for instance, the relaxation of the arteries of the skin in blushing, and the increased action of the heart in anger.[9]

Here was one of the first expansive works on a biological understanding of mind and body, and their interrelationship via the autonomic nervous system, which would be at the heart of Weekes' own work. Yet as far as the scientific canon was concerned, her writing in this area was to suffer much the same fate as Darwin's. As Dr Allan Schore, from the Department of Psychiatry and Biobehavioral Sciences, UCLA, pointed out in 2013, the autonomic nervous system was ignored for 'much of the last century'. However, 'a paradigm shift' took place in recent times from cognition to emotion — a shift back into the body.[10] Schore was not the only one to note that biology and human affairs were intermingled in the 19th century but that 'the two aspects developed along separate tracks for most of the twentieth century'.[11]

Ten years after the publication of *The Expression of the Emotions in Man and Animals*, Darwin died, aged 73. Yet the title of this 19th-century book identified an ambition still interrogated today: how can emotions be regulated? Implicit in this work was the idea of a collaboration between the mind and the body, that there was a commonality of emotional expression in humans and animals, implying they arose from those older parts of the brain that had developed early as survival mechanisms and were beyond conscious control.

Weekes' work was conducted under the giant umbrellas of the dominant intellectual influences of both Darwin and Freud. In a small way, her career would mirror these two giants. All three began as biologists, all started with an interest in evolution in animals, and all went on to investigate human emotion, inspired by their own turbulent psychic oceans. They all recognised that the mind could be taken hostage with the collaboration of the body. They all studied the autonomic nervous system, that bit of the body that was out of human control. They understood, personally, the tricks it could play.

Weekes' eventual understanding and treatment of anxiety was enhanced by her evolutionary studies. As a biologist, she understood the animal nature of man, how the mind belonged to a body that itself was governed by a set of evolutionary dictates beyond conscious control. Running away from a threat, blinking at the sun, and fighting for breath when oxygen was short were innate. Fear and hunger, love and lust were often associated with overt behaviours that resisted human management. Survival in both animals and humans was supported by *involuntary* behaviours. These unconscious instinctive reactions were assumed to be functional.

Freud himself was captivated by Darwin's evolutionary theories, which 'strongly attracted me, for they held out hope of an extraordinary advance in our understanding of the world'.[12] It was Freud who observed that 'humanity had to endure from the hands of science two great outrages upon its naive self-love', the first being from Copernicus' revelation that the earth was not the centre of the universe, and the second from Darwin, who undermined man's own centrality by establishing a continuity with animals.

Free will or conscious intent played a lesser role in human emotional behaviour if man was an extension of the animal. And if Darwin carried biological determinism into the field of emotion then Freud raced even further ahead, suggesting 'that most of human behaviour was motivated by drives that were largely unconscious, and therefore not the result of "free will"'. It was Darwin 'who handed Freud the most powerful instrument — namely, evolutionary theory's stress upon the dynamic, the instinctual, and, above all, the nonrational in human behaviour'.[13]

When Freud further assaulted the idea of 'rational man', he ignited a firestorm of controversy. He reinforced human helplessness, arguing man 'is not even mastering his own house, but that he must remain content with the various scraps of information about what is going on unconsciously in his own mind'.[14]

Freud originally accepted that anxiety had a biologically inherited basis and noted its value in helping an individual survive.

Fear had a protective and useful function.[15] Yet, as one of his many biographers argued, Freud was highly ambivalent about 'admitting the true extent of his intellectual debt to the field of biology. Indeed, once he finally achieved his revolutionary synthesis of psychology and biology Freud actively sought to camouflage the biological side of this creative union.'[16]

Freud is often called 'the Darwin of the mind', having charted his own inner life, which he famously explored to discern the outlines of unacceptable sexual fantasies. He also saw parallels between man's struggle to understand himself and the Darwinian concept of struggle for survival. He used Darwin's identification of 'instincts' in human and animal behaviour in his search for answers to the evolution of the human mind. Yet Darwin's judicious observations over decades, across real oceans, and on real continents, had more empirical status than Freud's inner journeys. Decades later, this lack of empiricism would prove a problem for Freudians, and many aspects of his theories faded under closer scrutiny.

In *The Expression of the Emotions in Man and Animals*, Darwin concluded a book full of examples of animal and human emotional behaviours with what could have been advice to an emotional patient.

> The free expression by outward signs of an emotion intensifies it. On the other hand, the repression, as far as this is possible, of all outward signs softens our emotions. He who gives way to violent gestures will increase his rage; he who does not control the signs of fear will experience fear in a greater degree; and he who remains passive when overwhelmed with grief loses his best chance of recovering elasticity of mind. These results follow partly from the intimate relation which exists between almost all the emotions and their outward

manifestations; and partly from the direct influence of exertion on the heart, and consequently on the brain. Even the simulation of an emotion tends to arouse it in our minds.[17]

Darwin might have been 'the first psychologist', but William James, who wrote over 1400 pages exploring the relationship between the mind and the body, became popularly known as 'the father of American psychology'. The brother of the famous novelist Henry James, he trained first as a doctor and then veered into psychology and philosophy at Harvard University, possibly drawn there by his own personal demons (his health was uncertain throughout his lifetime, and he suffered bouts of depression[18]). The result was his defining work, *The Principles of Psychology*, published in 1890. In 2018, his approach was described as 'strikingly modern'.[19] James declared that a genuine understanding of the mind–brain connection would constitute 'the scientific achievement before which all past achievements would pale'.[20]

In his own efforts to crack the code, James asked if it was possible to feel emotion without physiological arousal. He showed the interconnection, in the same way as Darwin had done in his final book. James wrote physiological psychology. He explicitly demonstrated how the nervous system primed the body without reference to conscious thought, and that emotions were often beyond control.

Fear was the primal example. Of all of the body's autonomic reactions, the unconscious threat response was unalterable. It was possible to control hunger, or even lust, but far harder to suppress the instinct to run from a charging bear. James memorably used the example of the bear, which was ridiculed by critics who thought he proposed that the running away was the fear itself. His work was then caricatured as suggesting that fear was nothing but the sensation of bodily changes, 'when all James meant to say was that bodily feedback was a necessary condition for emotion'.[21]

In 1894, James wrote that it would be impossible to think of the emotion of fear if 'the feeling neither of quickened heartbeats nor of shallow breathing, neither of trembling lips, nor of weakened limbs, neither of goose flesh nor of visceral stirring were present'.

Not everyone agreed. One scholar went so far as to assert emotion need not engage the body at all. The philosopher Ludwig Wittgenstein rejected the idea that the body needed to be involved. 'A man would say he grieves in his soul, not in his stomach, because you wouldn't expect to be cured of grief by relief from the unpleasant feeling in his stomach.' James surely would have disagreed with this, and Weekes certainly would. The fear that had taken her hostage as a young science student was felt expressly in her body — it was triggered by heart palpitations, after all. So what began with the autonomic nervous system was perpetuated by consciousness of fear, which in turn triggered an autonomic response. Thus the vicious cycle. James helped start the long unfinished argument about emotion. What was it, where was it, and of what was it composed?

In 1915, long after Darwin and five years after the death of James, the Harvard-trained American doctor and physiologist Walter Bradford Cannon took the science into the laboratory to understand how emotions were expressed in the body. He laid the foundations for somatic medicine with his experiments on the autonomic nervous system of cats and dogs, measuring exactly what happened to their hearts, lungs, digestion, and blood when they were alarmed. He elaborated on the mind–body connection, or, more accurately, the brain–body connection, in his publication *Bodily Changes in Pain, Hunger, Fear, and Rage: an account of recent researches into the function of emotional excitement.*

Above all, Cannon is remembered for his work on fear and its physiological source, the autonomic nervous system. He provided experimental proof of how the sympathetic nervous system, the brain's alarm centre, fired up the body. When frightened, or angry, the blood rushed to the key organs to prepare for what he unforgettably dubbed as 'fight or flight'. The heart raced, the breathing quickened, digestion was suspended, and the blood prepared to clot.

Graduating from medical school in 1900, Cannon was by 1906 the chair of the Harvard Department of Physiology and laid down more evidence of the mind–body connection, which would later get waylaid by psychoanalysis and the early schools of behaviourism.

Cannon's explorations of the sympathetic and parasympathetic branches of the autonomic nervous system reinforced the foundation of the biological view of stress and anxiety. Here was the feedback mechanism between the mind and the body that could lead to a better understanding of heart disease, digestive disorders, diabetes, and thyroid disorders — all deemed susceptible to stress.

Cannon's pathbreaking experiments involved monitoring gastric juices, sugar, and adrenaline in the blood of cats as they were terrified by dogs. It was the sort of work that Weekes' mentor Professor Harrison would have applauded — meticulous observation and measurement to support a theory. One of Cannon's chapters was titled 'Methods of Demonstrating Adrenal Secretion and its Nervous Control'. What Cannon showed was that, when highly aroused, the sympathetic nervous system pumped in the hormone adrenaline to prepare the animal for an emergency.

> The increase in blood sugar, the secretion of adrenin [adrenaline], and the altered circulation pain and emotional excitement have been interpreted … as biological

adaptations to conditions in wild life which are likely to involve pain and emotional excitement, i.e., the necessities of fighting or flight. The more rapid clotting of blood under these same circumstances may also be regarded as an adaptive process, useful to the organism. The importance of conserving the blood especially in the struggles of mortal combat, needs no argument.[22]

Cannon was later to become deeply engaged in exploring psychosomatic illness.

Taught to deal with concrete and demonstrable bodily changes, we are likely to minimise or neglect the influence of an emotional upset, or to call the patient who complains of that 'neurotic,' perhaps tell him to 'go home and forget it,' and then be indifferent to the consequences. But emotional upsets have concrete and demonstrable effects in the organism.[23]

He demonstrated the effect on all the major organs of the fight-or-flight instinct and had a neat metaphor for what could go wrong: 'One who commits fears, worries and anxieties to disturb the digestive processes when there is nothing to be done, is evidently allowing the body to go on to what we may regard as a "war footing," when there is no "war" to be waged, no fighting or struggling to be engaged in.' Completing the war metaphor in his last work, Cannon undertook to reveal 'how internal warfare may profoundly affect the whole organism and how return of internal peace may bring miraculously the return of health and happiness'.

Underlying Weekes' central theory of anxiety, and her treatment, was her biological understanding of the autonomic nervous system, and of the fight-or-flight reflex intimately implicated in the experience of fear. There were evolutionary 'built-ins' common to all living organisms. Fear had a purpose. A lizard would instinctively run away from a zoologist. She knew that that first intense flash of fear in the face of a bear, or any bear alternative, could not be suppressed or controlled in any way.

She too would use animal examples to make a point about the mind–body connection. 'Have you ever seen a frightened animal standing stock-still from fear or taking flight? Its nostrils and its pupils dilate, its heart races, it breathes quickly. The sympathetic division of the involuntary nervous system has prepared it for fight or flight.'

Darwin's book *The Expression of the Emotions in Man and Animals* inspired over a century of experiments on animals, in an effort to understand emotions in humans.[24] Yet a question hung over this work: did animals really feel emotions in the same way as humans? It was popularly assumed they did, and this belief justified experiments on animals, anticipated as providing a template for human treatment. However, the question of what emotional responses humans and animals shared remained controversial and there are now scientists who say it can never be proved.[25]

Animals can look frightened, terrified even, but do they suffer fear and anxiety in a way that is comparable to a human? Pharmacology has placed bets on the affirmative, and antidepressants are based on experiments with terrified rats. The question then inevitably is whether the results are transferable. The animal/human emotional analogy was challenged as far back as 1951,[26] and critiqued as recently as 2015 by the American neuroscientist Joseph LeDoux.[27]

Almost a century after the publication of Darwin's final book, Weekes married an evolutionary understanding of the mind–body connection with a more sophisticated understanding of the human brain. Understanding nerves meant understanding what was common to all animals, the primal survival response, and what was different. However, she stuck to a biologist's view of the mind and body, uninterested in the psychic speculations of Freud. By looking at the mind–body connection through the nervous system, she was an inheritor of the work of the 19th century, work that had been sidelined.

Weekes came to understand and manage her panic attacks, but whatever afflicted Darwin endured, and he withdrew from stressful situations, becoming very dependent on his wife, Emma, over the course of a lifetime for her calm and devoted support. Weekes, too, found a soulmate, possibly no less willing to protect and promote her genius than Emma was Darwin's.

The lesson Weekes would learn for herself and pass on to others was how to manage anxiety, of which a racing heart was just one manifestation. She aimed to show that while the heart was not always under the control of the will, it could come under the control of the individual. Her methods would change the history of treatment, and as Dr David Barlow has observed, to the unending benefit of tens of millions of people. Weekes was the first to identify the paradox that mastery over nervous illness is only achieved when control is totally relinquished.

Chapter 9

NOW, HERE WAS A TEACHER

The year 1929 was a personal turning point. Once Weekes understood she had been 'bluffed' by fear, she also appreciated that she had managed to complete her doctorate while shattered by nerves.

'While I suffered, I still worked. I submitted my thesis for my Doctorate of Science and got it. I can remember that while working my heart would bang heavily against my typewriter if I leant against it, but I still worked, I still did the thesis.' This was not just pride speaking. What had felt unbearable had been borne. The body proved stronger than she had believed, and she made this point in her books.

Beyond the 'simplicity' of Marcel Aurousseau's explanation of the fear suffered by soldiers in the trenches was his confidence in his diagnosis. His insouciance in the face of her distress was reassuring. This was another lesson. Confidence was contagious, and she had every reason to be confident in Aurousseau.

Weekes had needed Aurousseau's steadiness, and his first transforming words on fear fostered intimacy. They also now had mountains in common. Her UCL research required field trips, as she planned to study lizards at high altitudes in Europe to make comparisons with Australian skinks. Aurousseau knew the Pyrenees well, having crossed them in a long walk from Paris and Madrid, a journey he later turned into a book. He would be a perfect companion for her own explorations. At some point, the very tall, clever Aurousseau proposed to the very short, clever Weekes, and she accepted his proposal.

Aurousseau would point her in a new direction. The remarkable idea that fear had such power over the mind and the body reoriented her academic interests. Before leaving Australia, Weekes was already interested in neurology, or the study of the brain, and her curiosity now had a new, personal edge.

There was a significant opportunity in front of her in this respect, although it did not declare itself immediately. When she first arrived at UCL, Weekes had intended joining the experimentalists in her field of embryology, working with Professor James Hill and manipulating nature in the laboratory. She was also committed to further field research as she needed examples of pregnant lizards at high altitudes in Europe in order to buttress her cold-climate theory.

But by the late 1920s, Weekes' subject, zoology, was, like its partner, anatomy, losing cachet. 'The momentum of Darwin and Huxley waned; the scalpel and the injection needle grew rusty' as biochemistry and physiology were attracting many of the brightest students away from biology, and experimentation was in favour.[1]

Weekes was increasingly aware of the limits to lizards. She had achieved international recognition, but she had intensively studied these creatures for four years, two of which had been incredibly stressful, and the question was how much further she could take this reptile work. How much further did she want to?

Now she was back to her robust best, and she was elated. There were two sides to arousal and in place of dread she now had joy, of life, of travel, and of freedom from fear. Years later, she said she felt sorry for people who had never experienced nervous illness, perhaps because she knew the exhilaration of travelling down the other side of the mountain.

Before the year's end, in November 1929, and not six months into her course, Weekes looked over Dr Hill's shoulder, drawn to the force field of the head of the Department of Anatomy, the Australian Sir Grafton Elliot Smith, whose irreverence was more familiar to her than the formalities of English academic life, although she could be impressed by those.

Weekes continued her work with Hill, but, a year later, the records of the Rockefeller Foundation have an entry from W.J. Robbins' diary on her file card: 'is working with Prof.J.P. Hill. Will get advice of Prof.Hill and Elliot Smith before making final plans'.

Those plans presaged a complete redirection. Weekes was contemplating shifting from Hill to the 60-year-old Elliot Smith, not only a charismatic teacher, but one of the world's leading scholars of the brain. It was an irresistible combination. Anatomy may have been losing lustre, but the brain and nervous system were a different story altogether. According to one of Elliot Smith's friends and colleagues, Professor Frank Golby, the nervous system was 'the part of the body which was most in fashion, and which was attracting the most attention'.[2]

Like Weekes, Golby studied lizards but became disenchanted with their potential, particularly after he had experimented by removing the reptile brain only to find the animal was 'still, to all appearance, normal, except for a certain sluggishness'. Golby concluded that 'little is found in the brains of living reptiles to throw light on the evolution of the mammalian brain'.

Weekes was so galvanised by this opportunity to study the nervous system under one of the finest scholars on the subject, she was contemplating extending her studies at UCL and paying for Elliot Smith's course herself. If she wished to study the nervous system, she had little alternative as the Rockefeller Fellowship only ran for one year, and much of that was committed to fulfilling her lizard research promise to the foundation.

In the early 1920s, it was commonplace for scholars to play intellectual hopscotch, jumping from discipline to discipline, even if they had a specialty. One eminent scholar deplored the hastening trend towards specialisation in the early 20th century. 'Specialisation has in recent years reached such a pitch that it has become a serious evil. There is even a tendency to regard with suspicion one who betrays the possession of knowledge and attainments outside a narrow circle of interests,' warned W.H.R. Rivers,[3] a Cambridge scholar with a wide academic palette, including anthropology, neurology, psychology, and ethnology.

Contemporary scholars still voice the same complaint. 'In short, there is much to be learned and taught on all sides — but only if disciplinary boundaries can be overcome and the many different configurations of ideas can be related to each other.'[4]

In the Department of Anatomy at UCL, under Elliot Smith, Weekes was at no risk of being narrowed down. Regarded as the world's greatest comparative neurologist,[5] there was no better hurdler of academic boundaries than this large, compelling scholar and teacher whose own career trajectory began with the natural sciences, travelled to neurology, and from there to anthropology and psychology. He was not a man you could put in a box.

A biographical record of Elliot Smith recorded his intellectual athleticism: 'His mastery of cerebral morphology placed him, spiderlike, in the centre of the web of anatomical research, where acutely aware of movements in the measures, could sally with equal ease and rapidity to any part of its periphery. His many contributions to neurology, ophthalmology, psychiatry, psychology, zoology, and human palaeontology were as beads upon the connecting thread of his neuro morphological learning.'[6]

Elliot Smith believed biology offered insights into the mind and psychology.[7] In his early career, as professor of anatomy at Cairo University in 1900, he had been the first to X-ray the brains of about 6000 Egyptian mummies, which helped establish his authority on the evolution of the organ that especially separated man from other mammals. It was the 'mammalian nervous system, which remained, from boyhood to death, his abiding and absorbing interest'.[8]

This 'most vigorous controversialist' also demonstrated 'the ability to communicate plainly and intelligibly to the non-specialist the nature and fruits of abstruse biological research'.[9] It was a gift Weekes herself was to later demonstrate in her writings about anxiety.

Aurousseau took her to the crossroads and Elliot Smith led her down the path. Weekes had been her own personal experiment and had, with the help of her new fiancé, fixed herself. Now she was about be introduced to a biologist's view of the brain and the nervous system by a teacher who had the widest possible viewfinder on the experience of being human.

They had something else in common other than an interest in the mysteries of the mind. Like both Weekes and Aurousseau, Elliot Smith was passionate about music, and, like her, he loved to sing. Thomas Anderson Stuart, the Dean of Medicine at the University of Sydney who so disapproved of women studying medicine, had taught Elliot Smith physiology and remembered him as 'a very fine bass singer ... And if he had chosen an operatic career instead of an anatomical one he would have probably been equally successful.'[10]

Weekes was towards the end of her first year when she made a final decision to shift to neurology under Elliot Smith and his colleague, another Australian, Dr Una Fielding. There was more than just Weekes' new-found interest in the nervous system to consider, there was also Aurousseau. Returning to Sydney was not on the agenda.

Her Rockefeller records note that Weekes 'went over her change from J.P. Hill to Elliot Smith. W is sound in her view that in the remaining three months of fellowship she could only have taken up a minor problem in embryology, and that her allied problem in neurology could progress as well. Intends to stay on her own resources with Drs Felding [sic] & [Elliot] Smith until October.1931.' The comments were signed with just initials, WET, by a man who summed up his opinion of Weekes in three words: 'She is excellent.'

Under Elliot Smith, Weekes enrolled in a course on the 'ductless glands', an anatomical term for what was later called the endocrine system, the body's chemical messenger based on the secretion of hormones. There was a link to her lizard studies in that the endocrine system played a role in reproduction, but it had a wider remit and it was the bigger picture that appealed to Weekes. The ductless glands, worked in tandem with the nervous system, the electrical messenger.

The idea that hormonal activity influenced the nervous system dated back to the work of the ancients. In the second century AD, the first modern experimental physiologist, the court physician to Marcus Aurelius, a Greek known as Galen of Pergamon, proposed that 'vital spirits' in the blood regulated human bodily functions, and that 'nerves' were the mediators between mind and body. However, this was a concept that got frozen in time, and 'medical science remained stationary at best from Galen to the Renaissance'.[11]

Elliot Smith's course taught Weekes some basic lessons she eventually incorporated, years later, in her first book. The unsteady course of scholarship on nerves meant that when *Self Help for Your Nerves* was published in 1962, it was credited with providing 'contemporary medical views of nerves'.[12] The second chapter was titled 'How Our Nervous System Works'. The voluntary nervous system controlled the movement of the limbs, head, and trunk, 'and we control it more or less as we wish, hence its name'.[13] Weekes identified its counterpart as the involuntary nervous system, which 'controls the internal organs — heart, blood vessels, lungs, intestines et cetera even the flow of saliva and sweat'. This involuntary system in turn consisted of two parts, the sympathetic and the parasympathetic, the first of which 'strengthens an animal's defences against the various dangers which beset it, such as extremes of temperature, deprivation of water, attack by its enemies'.

As Walter Bradford Cannon identified, the sympathetic nervous system was responsible for releasing adrenaline, key to the fight-or-flight instinct, which was essential for survival but a curse when over-employed. As Weekes put it, 'sympathetic' was a misnomer for someone in its grip. It was the role of the parasympathetic nervous system to hold the sympathetic nerves in check, and it was only when 'we are overwrought that the sympathetic nerves dominate the parasympathetic and we are conscious of certain organs functioning. A healthy body without stress is a peaceful body.'

Elliot Smith was no Freudian, and, although psychoanalytic techniques had been broadly employed for years, he deplored what he dubbed the 'new Science of Sexology', suspecting, according to one of his colleagues, that 'scholastic pedants and pseudo-scientific charlatans took refuge behind a quasi-scientific edifice which they labelled "Psychology" in order to pour out a stream of literature which Elliot Smith always regarded as veiled (and thinly veiled) pornography'.[14]

Given his attitudes, he made a point, when training psychiatrists, to direct them towards a biological understanding of the nervous system.

'For some years before I came to London, it was my custom to give the students working for the Diploma in Psychiatry yet another form of neurology which aimed at the elucidation of the functions of the brain as an introduction to the study of the morbid anatomy of the central nervous system,' Elliot Smith explained in his *Fragments of an Autobiography*.[15] From him, Weekes learned that 'the mere biologist, while discussing strictly biological issues can call attention to certain psychological implications of anatomical facts and comment also on their neurological aspects for the interpretation of the mind and its workings'.[16]

He taught her about the circuitry of fear, and gave her the first glimmerings of an intellectual understanding of what could go wrong when this useful alarm could not be turned off.

Chapter 10

A TEMPLATE FOR A BOOK

Sigmund Freud was nearly 60 years old when World War I broke out. Although it offered a masterclass in mental as well as physical suffering, Freud, unlike many of his contemporaries, did not volunteer to help treat the tidal wave of wounded. He did not see 'a single one of these men, spending the war years immersed in writing his abstract theoretical papers and the *Introductory Lectures*, analysing his daughter Anna, and seeing those private patients who could pay his fees'.[1]

Freud turned away from the possibility of war trauma and kept his gaze focused on early childhood experience, wedded to the psychic constructs he proselytised. All neuroses had a sexual causation, and the war did not change his mind. According to one of his biographers, several of his 'erroneous conclusions regarding the war neuroses ... unfortunately endured because they were associated with his name and prestige'.[2]

On the side of the Allies, British psychiatry was taking a different turn. The psychologist W.H.R. Rivers wrote that there was 'abundant evidence that pathological nervous and mental states are due, it would seem directly, to the shocks and strains of warfare', and explicitly denounced the idea that there was any

evidence of repressed sexual complexes being to blame.[3]

Even then, Freud was a hindrance to understanding the trauma that followed war, and the problem was shunted off the agenda for half a century, until shell shock was reborn and identified as post-traumatic shock syndrome in the late 1970s as Western governments grappled with the broken soldiers returning from Vietnam. Most striking was Freud's 'neglect of fear as one of the most persuasive and intense emotions experienced in battle'.[4]

While Freud stayed away from the war wounded, Elliot Smith and his colleague T.H. Pear were drawn in the front door. Unlike Freud, they saw fear. Overwhelming fear. Then they intuited something else: 'that complex but very real state, the fear of being afraid'. They also were struck by how the consequences of this could play out in the mind and the body. After two years treating shell-shocked soldiers, Elliot Smith had, typically, forged his own strong opinions on the subject of nervous illness and plunged into the psychiatric debate, sleeves rolled up.

In 1917, *Shell Shock and Its Lessons* was published. It was a passionate and urgent treatise arguing for a compassionate approach to the shell-shocked soldier and for postwar reform of the entire field of mental health.

The symptoms of soldiers suffering from shell shock, were no different, Elliot Smith and Pear argued, from those seen off the battlefield: 'For shell shock involves no *new* symptoms or disorders. Every one was known beforehand in civil life … They existed before the war and they will not disappear miraculously with the coming of the peace.'[5]

The lessons learned from treating soldiers in wartime were applicable in peacetime. Elliot Smith and Pear advised closing the asylums and replacing them with clinics attached to hospitals, to give doctors experience in treating the mentally ill. They were adamant that medical practitioners be re-educated in the relationship between the mind and the body. Most controversially, they argued nervous illness was curable if doctors took the right approach to treatment.

In his introduction, Elliot Smith anticipated a more modern attitude by identifying an 'unstable blend of apathy, superstition, helpless ignorance and fear with which our own country has too long regarded these problems'. He recommended a postwar cultivation of 'the science of the treatment of mental disorders'.

Attracted as they were to the work of the French pioneer of psychotherapy Jules Dejerine, 'who advocated simple emotional sympathy as the most effective form of treatment',[6] their booklet crashed into both official and popular attitudes to 'insanity, or mental weakness'.

Nothing had been learned from the earlier wars about treating soldiers or citizens with nervous illness, Elliot Smith and Pear critically observed. Their last words in *Shell Shock and Its Lessons* were: 'We have dawdled away half a century and more in comparative idleness. Now the war has taught us a lesson. Are we to forget it again?'

Yes, could be the only answer to the rhetorical question. *Shell Shock and Its Lessons* itself was first overlooked, then forgotten. The lessons were unlearned, and soldiers' mental suffering would go untreated and unacknowledged for decades. There would be another world war and countless conflagrations afterwards. It took a further 63 years for war trauma to be officially recognised and medically acknowledged.

Instead of being remembered for his early insights into shell shock, history more noisily recorded Elliot Smith as a dupe, or worse, in the unsolved Piltdown Man hoax. (This was a fossil forgery putatively providing the evolutionary missing link between ape and man, but which turned out to be composed of a human skull, the jaw of an orangutan, and the teeth of a chimpanzee.)

One doctor, however, attended to *Shell Shock and Its Lessons*. If there was any template for the work of Dr Claire Weekes, this was it. The evidence that Weekes had read this critical work was firstly in an exactness of attitude and approach to the subject of nervous illness in the books she published 50 years later and the one that they wrote in the middle of World War I. Secondly, there was the circumstantial timing.

Weekes was being taught the latest scholarship on the fight-or-flight mechanism and its relationship to the adrenal glands by Elliot Smith not long after discovering that shell-shocked soldiers experienced the same unsettling mental and physical symptoms that had so bedevilled her.

In the small Australian scholarly circles in London, Aurousseau would have been known to Elliot Smith. They had both been to Sydney University and both men had been friends with Launcelot Harrison. They had all served in World War I, albeit in quite different ways. It's possible Aurousseau had heard of *Shell Shock and Its Lessons* and pointed her towards it. Or perhaps Elliot Smith, inclined to give his students a broad lesson in the nervous system, had mentioned it himself.

Whether Weekes came across the book is unknown, and yet any reading offered uncanny echoes of her own later work. It began with medical science and affirmed her own experience of how fear could derange the mind and the body. It also offered a different and very positive view of the sufferer. This was unusual at the time and remained so.

Where the government saw cowards, Elliot Smith and Pear saw the brave. The most severe and distressing symptoms occurred, they asserted, in 'those patients whose past history shows that, far from possessing even the normal measure of timidity, had been noted for their "daredevilry" and had been specially chosen as dispatch riders, snipers and stretcher bearers in the firing line'. The soldier and war poet Siegfried Sassoon was one example, although he was unnamed.

'It is quite common to find among the patients suffering from shock senior noncommissioned officers who have been in the army 15 or 20 years and have stood this severe strain. Such men can hardly be called weaklings or "neuropathic".'[7]

Or, as Weekes wrote, years later: 'these are some of the bravest people I have known. They tackle things and they have almost nothing within themselves with which to tackle them.' On the latter point, Elliot Smith wrote, 'There are warring elements inside as well as outside him: he is trying to fight the enemy with an army which is mutinied.'

There was no credit given by Elliot Smith and his co-author Pear to 'men who seemed immune to fear of danger. To them we scarcely apply the adjective "brave". The brave man is one, who feeling fear, either overcomes it or refuses to allow it to prevent the execution of his duty.'

Their assured, teacherly tone and everyday metaphors in *Shell Shock and Its Lessons* were a mark of Weekes' own later style, although it was possible the authors shared an Australian preference for plain speaking. She certainly shared their conviction that 'psycho neurosis may be produced in almost anyone if only his environment be made "difficult" enough for him'.

Elliot Smith and Pear aimed at jolting the professionals and the public from the view that some people were more likely than others to go mad, and that nervous illness was incurable. 'The behaviour of the neurasthenic differs from that of the normal person only in degree,' the two scholars declared.

They rubbished popular notions that a soldier had 'lost his reason' or 'lost his senses'. This was 'a singularly inapt description of such a condition. Whatever may be the state of mind of the patient immediately after the mine explosion, the burial in the dug out, the sight and sound of his lacerated comrades, or other appalling experiences which finally incapacitated him for service in the firing line, it is true to say that by the time of his arrival in a hospital in England his reason and his senses are usually not lost but functioning with painful efficiency.'

Elliot Smith and Pear were scholars, but they had chosen to write for a general audience, as Weekes would deliberately do herself. In their introduction, they said they had been repeatedly asked 'both by members of the medical profession and the lay public, to write a simple non-technical exposition of the ascertained facts of that malady, or complex of maladies, for which we have adopted the official designation shell shock'. Weekes similarly explained her decision to write popular self-help books, when, as a scholar, she may have been expected to aim for a professional audience. She said she saw that the public need for understanding was so great.

Coincidentally, the two men bracketed the treatment of mental illness in the same category as tuberculosis. What the two conditions shared apparently was a widespread belief that they were inherited conditions, a weakness that had been passed on. Weekes had suffered both, and both conditions had been stigmatised, wrongly from the point of view of Elliot Smith and Pear, who debunked the idea that heredity explained everything. Weekes herself later expressly rejected the idea that depression was inherited. This was particularly provocative for mental disorders, as the asylum system rested on this assumption, and had powerful institutional advocates at a time when treatment was highly contestable.

In *Shell Shock and Its Lessons*, Elliot Smith and Pear made the case for a more 'psychological' view. The key, they argued, to short-circuiting a tragic outcome, incarceration, and labels of insanity was to catch the sufferers early and teach them how to cure themselves, through a clear explanation of their symptoms.

'Understanding' was a keyword. Elliot Smith and Pear wrote: 'Not the least of the successful work performed in the special hospitals during the war has been the dispelling of fear by helping the sufferer to understand his strange symptoms (many of which are merely unusual for the patient himself) and, in the light of this new self-knowledge, to win his own way back to health.'

Forty years later, Weekes wrote: 'Understanding nervous fatigue is the key to understanding the baffling experiences that make recovery from nervous illness so elusive — within grasp one minute, gone the next. Understanding is the forerunner of cure.'[8]

There were stylistic similarities between her work and theirs. They favoured words in italics or in bold — the very thing that the very first reviewer of Weekes' first book deplored as typical of what he disparaged as the self-help genre. Even more exactly parallel were some key phrases. Where Elliot Smith and Pear protested against the proposition 'Once a lunatic, always a lunatic', saying it was as 'brutal as it is unjustifiable', Weekes echoed them, almost exactly, years later in 1983 when, addressing the Fourth National Phobia Conference, she criticised what she identified as the psychiatric attitude to their patients: 'Once a weakling, always a weakling.'

They talked of nerves, and nervous disease, the very words she would use half a century later. And if she did not read their words, she certainly shared their point of view that doctors should know better than to 'concentrate their attention almost exclusively upon the bodily ills of their patients' given that many of them well knew that 'not a small number of the maladies which come under their notice are seriously complicated, if not dominated by mental factors'. She built her reputation on understanding anxiety that presented psychosomatically.

Elliot Smith and Pear, like Weekes, tried to show people how to cure themselves and, in doing so, offered those critical ingredients, hope and confidence. Yet it was their emphasis on fear that made their work so redolent of hers. 'It could not be overstated,' they argued, that many of their patients at Maghull Hospital, north of Liverpool, were 'quite sane, if conduct be regarded as the criterion of sanity; but they are growing afraid of the appearance of these abnormal phenomena and take them for signs of incipient — or, more usually perhaps, of established — insanity'.

Here the two men had identified the phenomenon Weekes was to make central to her diagnosis — fear of fear would be one of her most enduring insights into understanding, treatment, and cure. She was the first to point out that so-called agoraphobia was less a fear of the 'agora', or the outside world, but instead was a dread of the return of unbearable *feelings* associated with going out. It was fear of the feelings returning.

One of the greatest sources of breakdown that Elliot Smith and Pear identified was 'intense and frequently repeated emotion'. Weekes coined the word 'sensitisation' to explain to sufferers why they were invaded with such baffling and disturbing feelings. As Elliot and Pear put it, 'These disturbances are characterised by instability and exaggeration of emotion rather than ineffective or impaired reason.'

So what was the answer? How to treat people in the thrall of an emotional response? Doctors were the answer, medical doctors, according to Elliot Smith and Pear. *Shell Shock and Its Lessons* devoted a chapter to their argument that doctors needed a much better understanding of psychology and of the way in which the disturbances of the mind could result in disturbances to the body.

The two scholars believed confidence was all — and a well-trained doctor could provide this. They acknowledged the 'suggestive' work of Walter Bradford Cannon. 'We were not unmindful of the part played by the sympathetic system, the adrenals and the thyroid glands in the development of symptoms of "shell shock …"'

It was a medical model of psychological suffering, and, if

Weekes read their booklet, she would have seen how confidence in the 'efficiency of an advisor's ability' had been an essential factor 'ever since mankind first sought help from his fellows for his afflictions of body or mind. To be able to convince a patient that he is going to recover, and that medical advice will help towards that end is certainly not the least of the physician's qualifications.' It was on this basis that Weekes insisted her publisher give prominence to her status as a doctor on the jackets of her books.

In *Shell Shock and Its Lessons*, Elliot Smith and Pear had linked nervous symptoms to the continued suppression of emotions. They simply observed this; they suggested no way of correcting the problem. Weekes was to have an answer, a most unorthodox answer in her later prescription of acceptance of the symptoms. It was counterintuitive, and it was a lesson she learned from Aurousseau. The soldier was trained to fight; the nervously ill instinctively fought their distressing symptoms. Weekes would prescribe a laying down of arms, an end to battle.

Shell Shock and Its Lessons stopped at the doctor's door, the authors resiling from the task of spelling out the mind–body connection, as they had neither time nor space. Yet Elliot Smith and Pear recommended that someone else tackle this 'most fascinating problem', which included 'the mechanisms by means of which emotional disturbances cause the disorganisation of bodily functions'. To have embarked on this 'would have involved a far-reaching excursion into most domains of clinical medicine'.

They had not, they acknowledged, written 'a complete manual upon the therapy of mental disease', and they would have to leave that to someone else. Weekes would write exactly that 'manual' in 1962 as a medically trained doctor, explaining in layman's language how the nervous system worked and setting out in detail all the related bodily systems that could collaborate with intense emotion to deliver such strange symptoms and such intense distress.

Chapter 11

LIFE IN A COLD CLIMATE

After seven months in harness in the labs at UCL, and before she shifted to Elliot Smith, Claire Weekes interrupted her scholarship year to take a long break to travel with her friend Cecily Vance and her fiancé, Aurousseau. It was not entirely unrelated to work as she used the opportunity to collect lizard specimens in the Pyrenees, among other more congenial activities. Not only did she have the Rockefeller money, but she had received a grant from the Royal Society of London, which covered the cost of field research in the Auvergnes, Pyrenees, and French Alps.

Weekes was given approval to defer the second half of her fellowship, and, on 30 May 1930, she headed off for her first European jaunt, with plans to interfere with unsuspecting high-altitude lizards. By 31 June 1930, Elliot Smith was writing introductions to various academics who could assist her.

It was a timely break and possibly doubled as a celebration. Weekes had regained her mental and physical health, and, several weeks earlier, on 5 May, had been awarded by the University of Sydney, in absentia, a doctorate in science for her thesis, whose title embodied its ambition: 'Placentation amongst Reptiles and Its Possible Bearing upon the Evolutionary History of Mammals'.

In April 1930, *The Sydney Morning Herald* reported that 'Miss Weekes has the distinction of being the first woman to be awarded the degree of Doctor of Science at Sydney University. The examiners reported that her thesis was an original contribution of distinguished merit adding to the knowledge and understanding of zoology.' They even published a photo of Weekes, whom they referred to by her birth name as Hazel, which she still used formally.

The Newcastle Herald reported 'that Claire Weekes, who won the only doctor's degree "Dr of Science" will not be there to receive it, as she is already on her way to Europe'. Apparently, Weekes was 'impatient to discuss with other learned scientists her important discovery of placentation among reptiles. This is expected to have an important bearing upon the evolutionary history of mammals.'

Aurousseau's future was now built around Weekes. He had ample time on his hands in London, and one way of making himself useful was to plan trips to help a woman studying lizards at high altitudes. She and Vance were happy to work up a sweat. This was to be an adventure, not luxury travel, and they spent much of the time hiking or riding bikes. Travel, now undertaken with a light heart for the first time in years, made such an impression on Weekes, she later attempted to wrestle it into a career.

Europe had her in its grip, and Australian newspapers reported on the thrill of discovery. One social columnist said that 'Candidly, I envy them, for they have enjoyed what I want to do most, when my luck is in, and I go for a visit to Europe. That is to visit the fascinating villages that nestle at the base of the Pyrenees on the Spanish side of the border. These two [Vance and Weekes], during their visit cycled over most of Europe, and four times crossed the Pyrenees on foot.'

This was well-trodden terrain for Aurousseau, who took them to the small town of Jaca, in north-eastern Spain on the border of

France. Weekes learned in Spain how to travel on a budget. The two women discovered they could survive on just five shillings a day.

Full of renewed confidence, Weekes was now reordering her priorities and shifting her academic focus to the brain. Travel had also piqued her interest in languages, which were such a passion of Aurousseau's. She paid for a course in Swedish, and told Australian newspapers that she and Vance added to their linguistic knowledge by 'three languages and a bit'.[1]

As Weekes' vigorous enjoyment of life returned, her confidence in her future as a married woman began to wane. Her relationship with Aurousseau had been the cornerstone of her postdoctoral life, and he was the man who had returned her sanity as well as being someone for whom she cared deeply. Yet in managing to return her to robust good health, Aurousseau had also reinvigorated Weekes' wider interest in the world. Now there was more on her mind than settling down to look after a husband.

Weekes and Aurousseau would go on to share a lifetime of interest in music, travel, and writing. It would be the last, writing, that would deliver them their greatest career triumphs and satisfactions, and yet their enduring relationship would be reforged. Aurousseau had saved her from herself and Weekes was grateful, and never forgot it. This was a strong foundation for friendship but not inevitably romance, and, in any case, she had decided to return to Australia. Weekes broke off the engagement.

It was a difficult time for Aurousseau. His friend Bert Birtles wrote that it was for him 'a spiritually fallow period with no clear objectives', although Aurousseau 'thought deeply at the time of writing a novel about five dominant women'.[2] Perhaps it was intended as cathartic. His former fiancée had been one of these.

The Great Depression was now biting into daily life, and economic pressures put his literary ambitions on hold. Aurousseau turned back to science, securing a position in the Royal

Geographical Society, and he settled down to what he described as a 'grind of a job in Kensington'.

On 2 October 1931, exactly two years after arriving in London, Weekes completed her studies at UCL, and she and Vance spent the next six months travelling again in Europe. The two young women went north this time, to Scandinavia, where Weekes could use her new Swedish language skills. They rode bikes 'from one end of Sweden across Norway' until it was time to go home.[3]

They sailed on the British ocean liner the SS *Orsova*, and arrived in Sydney on 9 March 1932. Like Aurousseau, Weekes was forced to adapt to the times. Her life had been untouched by the tentacles of the Depression until this point. London exposed her to a broader, more cosmopolitan life.

The 1920s had kicked off a wave of postwar energy, spawning art, books, and fashion that reviewed Victorian public morality. D.H. Lawrence had written his explicitly sexual *Lady Chatterley's Lover*, reversing traditional notions of sexual dominance. It was privately published in Italy in 1928, the same year Jonathan Cape published *The Well of Loneliness*, the first lesbian novel, and both books enjoyed the same fate: there was a public outcry and they were banned for decades.

The symbols of the time were, as usual, fashion statements. In the case of the emancipated woman, short, cropped hair signalled independence of mind and provoked anguished public debate about the decline of femininity. Weekes would never be especially interested in clothes or fashion, yet she joined this modish trend, picking the most boyish of all, the Eton bob, or Eton crop.

Her hair was cut close to her head, shaved at the back, and she dispensed with the curls at the side. A large photo in Women's World in *The Sydney Mail* on 9 March 1932 closed in on a sensitive, watchful face with soft, rounded features framed by extremely short dark hair and large, expressive eyes. Apart from the pearls, it could have been a photo of a young man.

Her arrival in the Antipodes with the Eton bob was noted by the newspapers. Not only did she look different from the woman who left the country two years before, but she returned with a wider education in life and all that Europe offered in music and the arts. Gone were those 'future plans' cited in her application for a Rockefeller Fellowship — to return to teach zoology at the University of Sydney. Lizards and laboratories had lost their allure.

She had travelled to London to work with Dr James Hill on lizards and returned without him. Instead, she spoke only of 'research work done with Professor Grafton Elliot Smith'. She told the press she had specialised in 'neurology — the function of the nerves and of the ductless glands, and she hopes to continue this branch of study at the medical school'.

She was, apparently, not missing a beat. 'Dr Weekes lost no time in getting into her stride in Sydney, for she started work in the Medical School today, four days after landing. She is the only woman doctor to graduate in science from Sydney University.'[4]

That more than glossed over the truth. It was a challenging re-entry as the Depression ended her ambitions for an academic post in neurology. Jobs were now a luxury. The year Weekes returned was counted as one of the most difficult in the history of the University of Sydney by its then vice-chancellor. Government funds were cut by almost a quarter; all academic salaries were cut by 10 per cent.[5]

This was no time to be fishing for appointments in a new academic pond, and so Weekes was forced to resume her old position at the university in zoology, now inaccurately described in the newspapers as her 'pet subject'.

Weekes enjoyed her standing as a serious scholar with an international reputation, yet she was losing interest in her specialty. The often-thankless grind of research was captured by her contemporary Dr Ethel McLennan, another of the tiny cohort of Australian women with a doctorate in science. 'To take up research as one's life requires a dogged determination and a complete disregard of all the usual ambitions of life for fame and fortune. Research people never expect to have any money, and if fame comes to them, it is often by sheer accident. Hundreds of people spend their lifetimes merely in marking a hundred or so promising roads "No Thoroughfare," and "Blind Alley," for the guidance of those who follow after them.'[6]

Weekes had gone as far as she wanted to go down the lizard lane. Although she had an international reputation, she found research a lonely endeavour. The laboratory felt like a cage for a woman who hated solitude. The return to Sydney brought larger career questions in its wake, yet she had no options available other than zoology. The next three years spent reluctantly in the field, however, further burnished her reputation. She earned renown for her cold-climate theory, which proved a lasting contribution to evolutionary scholarship.

Her work inevitably attracted some dissent. Before she left London, Weekes was challenged by another scholar at the Annual Meeting of the Anatomical Society of Great Britain and Ireland in 1931. She had been invited to address the society and read a paper on 'factors determining viviparity in reptiles', referring to 'the influence of factors such as endocrine activity, climate and more especially variations in temperature and degree of humidity, in determining whether one group or another would be the viviparous or oviparous'.

She met resistance from a Dr Emil Zuckerkandl, who was 'not quite persuaded that climatic factors were the sole factors determining the condition'. He objected that the theory implied 'a peculiar linkage of heredity and environment'.[7] Why couldn't mutation be responsible, asked her interrogator, possibly implying

Weekes had been captured by the Lamarckian idea that there had been structural changes to the lizards as they lived with the cold. Weekes' mentor Harrison had admired Lamarck's scholarship, but the French biologist remained controversial (although his ideas have been re-evaluated by some in light of discoveries in what is now called epigenetics, the study of how environmental influences can produce heritable changes in gene expression without changing the DNA sequence).

Weekes judiciously stepped aside from the evolution wars and relied on her own work. If she were going to argue with champions in the field, she would save that for Sigmund Freud decades later. The society's minutes reported her saying there was no evidence of the conditions of oviparity or viviparity being determined by mutations, and that it would take many thousands of years for any species of animal to change its habits.

An inclination to credit environmental influences was evident in her attitude to mental health in later years. Many scholars adhered to the idea that depression was inherited, but she demurred.

'In my opinion, depression may not be inherited as much as caused by environment. The mood of one member of the family can be too easily flattened by the depressed attitude of another member,' she wrote in her fourth book. 'Also, if several members of the family suffer with depression, other members can too easily become afraid that they too will eventually suffer from it. A sure way to become depressed is to be constantly frightened ...'[8]

For over a decade, Weekes had collected lizards in Australia and Europe, ultimately proving that they were predominantly live-bearing high above sea level. This pattern was confirmed repeatedly, and she identified three different placental stages, which she outlined in detail, 'revealing "unsuspected sophistication and diversity"', according to Professor Richard Shine, writing in this field almost a century later.[9]

By 1935, she had written the last of eight papers for the Linnean Society of New South Wales, in which she concluded that simple barometric pressure was unlikely to be the direct cause of viviparity, given that some sea snakes evolved as live-bearers at sea level. 'It seems more plausible that if there is an external factor associated with high altitudes influencing the adoption of viviparity, then that is cold, whether working by directly interfering with the oviparous cycle or by merely supplying conditions under which some mutations towards viviparity can work best.'[10]

She cited the geckos — subtropical and egg-bearers in the main. Yet in cold New Zealand, geckos had been found to be viviparous, which supported her theory. Live-bearing lizards were found exclusively at higher altitudes — above 4000 feet — and the lizards she'd studied across continents in varied alpine habitats confirmed her thesis that in cold weather lizards tended to retain their eggs for longer. She then tentatively prodded for a place in evolutionary history, arguing it was 'conceivable that the mammalian yolk sac placenta could have evolved along lines similar to these'. Her final paper was cited hundreds of times in subsequent academic work in the field. Exactly 80 years after her last paper was published, Weekes was still celebrated by contemporary zoological scholars.

> Weekes' (1927a, b, 1929, 1930, 1935) contribution to an understanding of reptilian placentation is monumental. She championed a comparative approach to the study of evolutionary patterns and generated hypotheses that remain relevant and are now subject to test within phylogenetic frameworks. Her work has had a dominant influence on more recent research of reptilian placentation both as a theoretical foundation and because she identified species that have continued to be useful models.[11]

Between 1931 and 1935, as Weekes ploughed on with her lizard research, she was in demand as a public speaker. She enjoyed the recognition, and she would retain her status as the only woman in New South Wales with a Doctor of Science degree until 1938. Yet when she was invited to address public audiences, she preferred to talk about travel, which had a wider appeal than placentation in lizards.

What was privately apparent, but not publicly known, was that Weekes was restless at the university. She had lost interest in Aurousseau as a husband, and now she was tiring of academia. If Weekes was unsettled, however, her closest friend was shaken. Proximity to Aurousseau had had an awkward outcome — Vance had fallen in love.

This was problematic, but not for the obvious reasons. Weekes told a number of different stories over the years about her attitude to her failed romance, all of which suggested that she was completely happy to leave her former fiancé to Vance and that she even ushered Vance towards him. The problem for Vance was not Weekes, but the object of her desire. When Vance hurried back to England to re-establish contact, Aurousseau remained blithely unaware of her interest in anything more than a friendship. He would keep the blinkers on for a decade.

Weekes later gave a couple of versions of her engagement to different nieces, telling Frances that, despite being very much in love with him, she had decided to 'give' Aurousseau to her great friend. She said she had made this sacrifice because her friend was besotted. Frances was not entirely convinced. 'Aunty could play the martyr at times. She said to me, "Well, you know Suze was so in love with him that I stood back."'

Standing back was not Weekes' modus operandi when she wanted something, and a slightly different version of her decision was given to another niece. 'She said she was engaged once,' Lili Louez recalls, 'and I remember her telling me she was very much in love with this man, and he was very much in love with her, and he married one of her friends.' Yet Lili remained baffled. She further interrogated her aunt: she would have made a wonderful mother; did she never consider children? This time, Lili got a different take. Weekes was clear that she regarded marriage as very much a second choice. Her career, she said, came first.

'"Do you know, darling, I dedicated my life to medicine. That was my first love — I just loved medicine and science, and, had I married, I would have been a wife, and I would have had to have been the best wife because I wanted to be the best at medicine." I will never forget her saying that,' says Lili.

This was factual, if incomplete. Weekes certainly wanted to be the best at whatever she was doing. She understood the quest for perfection and its emotional cost. She later counselled that too often aiming for the immaculate life was counterproductive. She would know. Being good, being the best, had a price. She was also quite truthfully admitting that striving to be the best wife would have sabotaged a brilliant career.

Chapter 12

THE SONG OF BETH

Weekes turned 30 in 1933. She was stuck in the zoology department and straining for a new direction beyond the boundaries
of her specialisation. While she was considering her next career
move, she took up an old family passion, music, enrolling in part-
time singing lessons at the NSW State Conservatorium of Music.
She loved German lieder, and 'the Con' had been founded with
the express aim of 'providing tuition of a standard at least equal to
that of the leading European Conservatoriums'.[1] This was to be a
life-changing decision.

Music was part of the family legacy. Many of the Weekeses
were musical, and, while she did not play an instrument, Weekes
had a fine singing voice. Vaudeville, very popular at the turn of
the century, had been her father Ralph's mainstay, and he played
both the violin and the drums for the profitable Harry Rickards'
Tivoli orchestra as well as for the well-known impresario J.C.
Williamson. Ralph was 'popular, wore bow ties and had bohemian artist friends', so, along with her mother, Fan, bashing away
on the keyboard, 'there always seemed to be something musical
happening', her brother Brian recorded in his memoirs. Fan loved
to play, but the ever-critical Brian remembered 'in my cruel way'

that she was a bit of a musical thumper. He dubbed her style 'Mum's Wash Tub touch', but conceded that 'she didn't hit wrong notes and enjoyed the music lots more than Dad!'

Yet it wasn't all musical slapstick and catchy tunes, as Ralph Weekes also played for the Sydney Symphony Orchestra and turned his hand to musical composition, the results of which won modest praise in the local newspapers, along with the odd sneer. While his 'April Showers' 'had been played with success at the Theatre Royal and the Town Hall',[2] his 'Love's Welcome' was damned by one critic who suggested he had written music to match the words he was given, which were 'of the ultra-sentimental order, and demand a sort of feeble prettiness. The music therefore could hardly be appropriate without being commonplace, and it is quite appropriate.'[3] Not every reviewer was as damning with one describing it as 'a pretty drawing-room ballad'.[4]

By the time she was in her 20s, Weekes had an extensive interest in, and grasp of, classical music, enhanced by her European travels. The Con trained serious musicians but also offered singing lessons on a part-time basis. A singer must breathe well, and the scientist in her understood that the breath was the one autonomic function of the nervous system over which some control could be maintained. Breathing could be slowed down. The nose or mouth employed. A deep breath could be taken, a longer exhalation practised. An understanding of physiology could improve technique.

A singer needed an accompanist, and Weekes acquired one of the Con's best teachers of pianoforte, Elizabeth Coleman. Coleman was four years older than Weekes and an acclaimed pianist. Taller than the tiny Weekes, she was a practising Catholic with a keen sense of propriety.

Popularly known as Bessie Coleman, she had her own substantial career, and to Weekes' modest file of newspaper cuttings she had an entire folder. She had been singled out as a protégé by the Con's founding director, the Belgian conductor and violinist Henri Verbrugghen. Appointed in 1915, he gave her 'special interpretation lessons' and she was for many years an accompanist to the Conservator in Choir under his baton.

An early photo in the local paper under the headline 'Con's Best Pupils' captures a solemn, well-sculpted face, a brunette with a romantic, dark-eyed melancholy. According to the newspaper report, Bessie Coleman played Beethoven's Piano Concerto No. 3 in C minor for her diploma test with the State Orchestra. 'Miss Coleman has a special gift in classic interpretation. She is a Sydney girl and belongs to a family of journalists.'[5]

The daughter of 'Mr FJ Coleman of Chatswood, a well-known Sydney Pressman'[6] attracted attention early in life. Her musical talents were first mentioned in 1909 when one newspaper reported on 'a much-boomed young Lassie in Sydney ... Little Miss Bessie Coleman who, in her 10th year, has passed the examination for Associate of the London College of Music obtaining 89 marks.'

By 1920, the 'chief interest' at a concert by the Conservatorium Orchestra at the town hall 'centred on the playing of this Bessie Coleman, whose interpretation of the Schumann in A minor was exceedingly clever'. The next year, she was 'one of the finest flowers of our Conservation Nursery',[7] and she was appointed as the professor of pianoforte there, having attained a Teachers and Performance Diploma.[8]

By 1924, there were more favourable reviews. 'Miss Bessie Coleman's pianoforte solo revealed that lady as a technician of high attainments. In addition, she possesses that somewhat rare quality — the gift of artistic expression and "soul"'. Miss Coleman in addition to her excellent soul 'rendered admirable service as an accompanist'.

The two women formed an immediate and rewarding collaboration, with Weekes singing the classics to Coleman's fine accompaniment. It was not long before they had renamed each other — Claire called Bessie 'Beth', who in turn called her 'Clara'. The experience was sufficiently profound to turn Weekes' attention in an entirely new direction. Singing lessons increasingly took up more of her time, although she had kept up her day job in the University of Sydney's zoology department.

For Weekes, this offered a higher education in music. It was also a joy. Over three years, the rapport built between the singer and the pianist was such that Weekes saw a way out of academia. With her newborn confidence, in herself and her talented partner, she decided that music would be her career, her future.

Weekes valued her standing as a Doctor of Science even as she was tiring of research and the lonely laboratory work — but the excitement of the stage, the rapture of song, and this satisfying collaboration with Coleman triggered a determination to pursue not just an entirely new, artistic career, but an international one at that. Weekes now planned to become a professional singer, and she harnessed Coleman to her venture. She would be launched on Europe's stage, with the help of her accompanist.

Prepared as she was to slam the laboratory door, Weekes was jealous of her status as a scientist, so she worked out a way of lashing her academic standing to her new venture. Having studied the physiology of breathing in anatomy, she decided she would not only sing but could teach singing from a 'scientific' perspective. The 'science of singing', she dubbed it.

Many years later, as a doctor, Weekes trained asthmatics in proper diaphragmatic breathing, including her niece Tita, who credited her with retraining her breath and thereby straightening out her rib cage. Over-breathing was implicated in high anxiety, resulting in oxygen overload with all its physiological side effects.

As a doctor, and then as a writer, Weekes later offered practical advice on slowing the breath that many found helpful, including

Les Murray, one of Australia's best-known poets, who suffered for years from debilitating depression. Murray eventually wrote a book about his experience of depression in which he attributed 'a simple breathing technique, from Dr Claire Weekes's writings, which got rid of the tingling in my fingers by reducing the acidity of my blood. This acidity results from overbreathing, sucking in an excess of air in preparation for a battle or a panic flight that never happens.'[9]

Weekes and Coleman planned their trip to Europe, where both had connections they hoped to translate into opportunities. Weekes' two brothers, Brian and Alan, inspired by Weekes' success abroad, had tried their own luck and were now living in London themselves. Despite the global depression, both were employed by multinational advertising agencies, jobs that set them up for life. Fan attached herself to the adventure, as did Dulcie, and they headed to London together. Ralph was left home alone.

The local newspapers reported their departure, recording the achievements of the two professional women. 'Dr Claire Weekes and Miss Elizabeth Coleman left by the Ormonde on May 25 to further their studies abroad. Dr Weekes won the Rockefeller scholarship several years ago, and after remaining abroad for three years returned to Australia to resume her science research as a Macleay fellow. Miss Coleman is a well-known pianist and tutor at Sydney Conservatorium, and she was entertained by other members of staff at a farewell party. Both the travellers are looking forward to being present at the Salzburg Festival. Mrs F Weekes, Dr Weekes' mother and her sister Dulcie will also travel to London by the Ormonde to visit Mrs Weekes two sons, Mr Alan Weekes, who is a writer, and Mr Brian Weekes, an artist.'

The *Ormonde* passed through the port of Fremantle on the other side of the country, and local newspapers were attentive. The Perth *Daily News* published a photo of the two women, with a rather severe bespectacled and hatted Weekes sitting with a relaxed-looking Coleman in a cloche hat standing behind her. The newspapers had been well briefed about Weekes' ambitions. The headlines included 'Science of Voice Production. Dr H.C. Weekes' Mission' and 'Doctor of Science to Study Singing'. Weekes was described as 'a slim alert Australian' who said her decision to study singing 'was no revolutionary feminine reaction, but the outcome of a lifelong ambition'.

Weekes presented her new career experiment as an extension of her academic path. 'I have been doing scientific research, specialising in glands,' she said, 'and now I'm going to study the physiology of voice production. After all singing is a science.'[10]

The Bessie Coleman of yesterday had become her 'friend Elizabeth' in the newspaper reports, which noted the pianist had 'encouraged' Weekes and played her accompaniments at the Conservatorium. They were bound for the Salzburg Festival in Germany, then Vienna, and were planning to be away for three to four years, according to Weekes, who regarded England not just as a place to visit but as a great jumping-off point for the rest of Europe. Australians, she said, spent far too much time visiting 'home'.

Their schedule was packed. Weekes was an ambitious traveller, and the two women spent time in the Netherlands, Belgium, France, Italy, Germany, Austria, and even Czechoslovakia. Music was never far from their itinerary, and they knew the hometowns and homes of every famous composer, and could critique in detail, down to the violins, the many concerts they saw. Their trip was followed closely by the press back home. *The Australian Women's Weekly* had a small item dedicated to Coleman. The headline: 'Pianist for England'.

When they eventually arrived in London, Weekes' two brothers, Brian and Alan, were at the wharf to greet them. Fan's sons were reminded immediately of their mother's stubborn

eccentricities. Brian later told his children of his horror at the sight
of Fan marching down the gangplank accompanied by her own
mattress, which had travelled with her from Sydney.

That period in London was about the last time that Fan's
youngest son spent much time with his mother. Before too long,
the urbane Alan married a woman he regarded as a class above his
own mob, and he stepped aside from the Weekeses, the occasional
exception being his elder sister.

Weekes was never as close to Alan as she was to her other
siblings, despite the fact that they shared restraint in common, the
very quality missing in Brian. It was the noisy, troubled Brian who
would cleave to Weekes despite all their obvious differences. Brian
once described his clan as being streetwise. 'All the bloody Weekes
were! I just don't know what street …'

The trip was entirely satisfactory from a travel point of view.
Fan and Dulcie stayed with them for one year, and, at some stage,
Coleman's mother also joined the travel party. The trip was
increasingly taken up with sightseeing as it soon became obvious
that only one of them was going to make it in Europe — and that
was Coleman, whose reputation in the field preceded her and led
her to one of the most famous European sopranos of the day,
Elisabeth Schumann.

Born in Germany, Schumann had performed in the Hamburg
Opera, and then in New York before becoming the star of the
Vienna State Opera from 1919 to 1938. By the time Weekes
and Coleman arrived, she had long been a fixture at the annual
Salzburg Festival. The vivacious, elegant Schumann was closely
connected to all the leading musicians of the day, including
Wilhelm Furtwängler, Otto Klemperer, and Richard Strauss.
Married three times, Schumann left her first husband for the
brooding Klemperer, who became just another in a long line of
men she loved.

In a significant tribute to Coleman's talent, Schumann had her as accompanist on the piano in three of the soprano's *Schubert Songs*, which was recorded in London at Abbey Road Studios. For Weekes, it was a mixed experience. Coleman was living up to expectations, but she had arrived with provenance. Weekes was starting from scratch, with a reputation as a scientist to 'sell' herself, but without any professional brand.

She saw for herself that she would be competing with the likes of Schumann, who, as a famous soprano, also taught singing and breathing technique. Schumann had a fine voice, but it was not as strong as other contemporaries, thus her interest in the breath.

The pleasure of seeing Coleman succeed, and hearing her matched with the voice of Schumann, must have amplified Weekes' own failure to get any traction. However, travel offered other consolations.

In Salzburg, they visited the 'quaint Mozarthauschen, a tiny house in which Mozart wrote the score of The Magic Flute'. They went to Versailles, spent a few months in London, and visited Vienna twice.

The newspapers in Sydney were reporting it as Coleman's trip.[11] Music was the main theme given the women's professional intentions. The papers reported that she attended a program of Beethoven's music 'given in the courtyard of the Beethoven house; another of Schubert's works, given in the house where this composer was born; and an open-air choral recital of 2000 voices, given in front of the Town hall'.[12] And she 'was in the Austrian capital during the festival week, which always brings forward a fine array of musical and dramatic events. Singers at the State Opera camp in Stockholm, Prague, Budapest and New York.'[13]

Weekes was relegated to companion status but kept herself busy writing detailed notes of her travels. The daily tabloid *Truth* newspaper wasn't buying the science angle and just reported that

Weekes 'has abandoned science pro tem and is having her lovely singing voice trained'.[14]

Part of Weekes' record of her trip was later published in the *Newsletter* of the Women's College at the University of Sydney. It revealed the depth of her immersion in music: 'So far Furtwangler and Mengelberg have made the deepest impression as conductors — Toscanini for Mozart opera but for Beethoven and Brahms, Mengelberg and Furtwangler have a breadth of treatment that I cannot find in Toscanini or many other conductors for that matter.'[15]

It was not just the music that held her attention but the technical performance of the players. She noted a violinist 'with a marvellous technique. His fault was born from his virtue. His bow moved so easily that it sometimes pressed too heavily and attacked too forcibly, and the tone was spoilt. His rhythm too, was excellent although his Tchaikovsky playing was a little too refined but Mengelberg always brought the orchestra in with just that touch of savagery the Russian needs.'

As the months marched on, dreams of a shared musical career with Coleman slowly died. Weekes would never teach singing yet remained fascinated with the voice, and, decades later, Paul Skene Keating, the son of one of her closest friends, believes she was well ahead of her time, and his recollection is that she learned from Schumann herself. Weekes was, he says, 'incredibly knowledgeable' about the voice. 'Having the medical background as well as the mechanics, and understanding the function, meant she was riveting on the subject.'

She understood the importance of correct breathing, correct posture. Skene Keating recalls her explanation that most people shallow-breathed, almost from the chest, 'and that the breath should come from the bottom of the lungs so that your abdomen actually swells out widely and then you get maximum capacity of air into the lungs.' Think of how you can hear a baby screaming blocks away, literally. 'We talked about that a lot, and that was long before people came to acknowledge that.'

Weekes retained a lifelong love of music, but this fledgling career was soon on hold. At some stage, she recognised that she did not have what it took to either make singers or be one herself.

The two women had planned to stay away for three to four years but instead returned after just two on the cruise ship *Awatea*. They landed in Sydney on 8 January 1937, and the newspapers were ready to report on these 'two brilliant young Sydney women'. Coleman ranked first in the report, ahead of Weekes, who, with no successes of her own to broadcast, directed her communication skills in the service of Coleman's collaboration with Schumann.

Her pride in her friend was obvious, and she didn't miss the opportunity to underline Coleman's achievement in accompanying the famous European soprano. 'This was a great honour,' said Weekes, 'for Madam Schumann has never been accompanied by a woman, and never by an Australian.' Weekes pointed out it was more than just a professional engagement but had evolved into a friendship. The newspaper duly reported the details. 'They were frequent visitors to her flat in Vienna and were invited to her Bavarian chalet for the summer ... here she has a large music lounge room with a grand piano, a wireless set, and a complete set of her own recordings.'

Coleman was interviewed, and proffered the following opinion on Schumann: 'she is a sweet person and is always singing about the house and in the garden. We heard her in Mozart and Strauss's operas in Vienna and Lieder recitals in Amsterdam and London. Her favourite composers are Schubert, Mozart and Strauss.'

For a while, Weekes stuck to the singing script, although *The Sydney Morning Herald* seemed far more interested in her 'Folding Umbrella from Paris', with its flexible ribs, and they used this headline over a large behatted photo of her accompanied by shots of her opening and shutting it. They also liked her navy spotted 'swagger coat with a Peter Pan collar'. 'Although Ms Claire Weekes D.SC, treats even singing seriously and scientifically, she has an appreciative eye for smart frocks and accessories,' it opened.[16] She did love coats, it was true, and later bought a couple in lamb's wool, so large that only her head and lace-up shoes emerged from their cavernous interiors. However, this was possibly the first and last time Weekes was offered up as a fashion exemplar.

Mostly, the press asked her about her singing 'science'. 'While Miss Coleman made her first trip abroad merely as a holiday to absorb and enjoy music, Dr Weekes went with the definite intention to study the physiology and physics of singing, to equip her later to "make singers."'

This 'outstanding pupil of Sydney Girls High School' who had a 'brilliant career doing research in science at the University of Sydney' described her studies abroad as 'a form of scientific research', according to the newspaper. Yet Weekes knew this 'research' was leading nowhere, although she did not publicly announce its demise. Instead, she unveiled a new career plan, again completely unrelated to everything that had gone before, and even more startling than her abrupt switch from research on lizard placentation to singing on the world stage.

'She has travelled extensively in Europe, and while she is completing her studies Dr Weekes intends to open a European Travel Advice Bureau in the city, planning whole tours economically,' the paper reported. It was another career somersault. Weekes was not afraid of change, nor modest in her ambitions as she hankered, in all her ventures, for an international stage. There was no sign of the bewildered young woman she had been, and there was a new steadiness in her life, which could be attributed to her relationship with Coleman.

At home, however, there were significant adjustments to be made, the main one being that the two women were separated for the first time in two years. According to *The Sydney Morning Herald*, 'Miss Coleman' was returning to her parents, Mr and Mrs F.J. Coleman of Chatswood, and 'Dr Weekes' would stay with her sister, Mrs Muir Maclaren, at Darling Point. Dulcie at this stage was married and about to have her first daughter, Frances, in 1938.

However, this female diaspora was not to last. Fan did not want to let go of her girls, and Weekes and Coleman wanted to live together. It would take a little time, but eventually Fan's girls would be gathered together — and stay together for their lifetimes.

Chapter 13

DR WEEKES' EUROPEAN TRAVEL ADVICE BUREAU

For the next two years, Weekes did not take a weekend off.[1] Her work ethic, which had always impressed her mother, sometimes irritated other members of the family. Weekes had priority, and Fan would remind anyone who forgot of the needs of the favourite child. 'Sshh, Claire is working, or sleeping' was the regular refrain, from the vigilant parent.

There was a real urgency to the task in front of her. Although Weekes did not look back with any regret to her years in science or academia, she was now starting over again at the age of 35 years. She wanted a new career, and she wanted to be the 'best', as she put it. A period of unemployment was no immediate threat as she was single and had some economic flexibility. She could always stay at home, where she was indisputably the premium family product.

Still, there was pressure to succeed in the Weekes family, and to conform as well. All the children felt it, and Brian with his medley of gifted and discordant traits twisted wildly within the family straitjacket. In a letter to his daughter Barbara, written years later in 1985, Brian lamented his parents' expectation that they all be 'carbon copies of their upbringing'. It was 'soul destroying cater-pillarism, one exactly following the other', he wrote. 'No Weekes will ever bludge on his or her job — we fear failure too much'.[2]

On 18 December 1937, *The Australian Women's Weekly* reported on her travel bureau. 'Dr Weekes has lived and studied in Europe for many years. She was impressed by the possibility of Australians travelling in Europe much less expensively than is commonly believed and is now aiming to teach them how to do so.'[3]

If Weekes' abrupt abandonment of a stellar career in scientific research had seemed impulsive, her new travel gambit was even more quixotic. She had worked up a scheme to buttress the proposed travel bureau by becoming a newspaper columnist, having watched others make words their living, albeit with mixed results. Aurousseau had written travel books, although this never offered an income, and Amy Mack had built a reputation as an expert on the Australian bush through her newspaper articles. Moreover, Weekes had 'connections' in the press.

As for travel, Weekes believed she knew more about it than most Australians and noted that even those with experience tended to cleave to Great Britain. She was leaning away from safe and serious professional choices towards what she actively enjoyed and was proceeding in quite experimental directions with utter confidence. Her tolerance for uncertainty was buffered by a happy private life.

She understood she could not live on writing alone, but a newspaper column that identified her as an expert would be an effective marketing tool to promote her bureau. *The Sunday Sun and Guardian*, a Sydney tabloid established in 1929, servicing the largest capital-city market in Australia, was then one of Australia's most successful newspapers, with a circulation of over 250,000.[4] It could deliver a broad audience.

Her brother-in-law, Muir Maclaren, was a journalist, but the man who would prove the key contact was Beth Coleman's father, Fred, the state reporter on *The Sunday Sun*. With some persuasion, Weekes soon got her weekly column.

Her proposed business had three arms. The first two would work hand in hand. The column would help publicise her bureau in Sydney, where all information regarding travel in Europe could be obtained. Finally, she would make money from international visitors. She had identified a gap in the travel-advice market for what she called a 'comprehensive official guide book of Australia for the overseas tourist'. It was to be 500 pages long and would be modelled on the famous Baedeker Guides, which had dominated the market since the mid-19th century and upon which she had relied extensively in her own travels. The book would be completed by late 1939, and she planned to travel the length and breadth of the Australian continent to research and write it.

Weekes told *The Australian Women's Weekly* that she was 'writing the backbone of the book herself' but contracting with experts on various subjects, such as the South Australian wine industry and the early history of Adelaide. 'It will be a complete guide,' she promised.

With the same bravado that had propelled her previously determined pursuit of international success, Weekes told the newspapers, too, 'It will be in circulation all over the world; in fact, I am hoping to have it ready for sale at the World Fair in New York.'

A bit like selling 'singing as science', this project had its own special challenges, Australia's distance from overseas markets to begin with. For the next two years, without a day off, Weekes wrote her weekly column, researched the guidebook, and simultaneously lobbied anyone who could supply information for her book or fund her business venture, either with cash or by paying for advertising. As she travelled, she made presentations to local councils, tourist agencies, shipping companies, and state governments.

Her subject, Australia, was complicated by scale. The sixth largest country by size and the world's biggest island continent, it offered more geography than history or tourist culture. The language was more or less the same from Sydney to Perth, a distance of over 3000 kilometres. There wasn't even local argot. Insofar as there was any appreciation of the culture maintained throughout the centuries by the downtrodden Indigenous Australians, it would not gather mainstream interest for generations. At that time, native Australians had no voice, no vote, and no respect.

Whatever Australia had going for it in the tourist market, it was not the Antipodes' answer to Europe. If Australians left the city, they were 'going bush'. There were lovely beaches, but it was a long way to go for a swim, and there was no popular market for environmental tourism. Australians were known for having 'a chip on their shoulder', meaning that they felt inferior.

Weekes understood the magnitude of her task. 'Romantic histories and Australian settlements are not so abundant that we can afford to pass one by,' she told a reporter in 1939.[5] It was easier to write about Europe than identify Europe in Australia, which she strained to do in her guidebook. She wrote of inns in small coastal towns in NSW that somehow reminded her of those in England. It must have been a relief to reel off her weekly *Sunday Sun* column about travelling in Europe, with its rich tourist offerings, for Australians.

Her column aimed to 'help Australians to travel abroad economically'. *The Sunday Sun* launched her 'unique Travel Service', inviting readers to write to Dr Weekes, who would 'help you plan your tour of Europe'. She told the Adelaide *Advertiser* that she had a more thorough knowledge of Continental cities, and how to travel 'at considerably less cost', because she had made most of her own journeys 'on foot or by bicycle'.

Her first column, Weekly Travel Service No. 1, was published on 16 January 1938, and Weekes sounded the trumpets: 'The age of travel as the prerogative of the plutocrat is over.' From this democratic platform, she launched what would be almost 100 columns. She would write one a week, every week, for two years. This 'brilliant' scholar, with a doctorate in science and a vernacular honed in the earthy Weekes-family household, did not need to be taught how to write for a popular audience. It was 'possible to live comfortably in London on 5-pound sterling per week without undue economy', she reported.

Weekes made a point of including her gender in this egalitarian travel revolution. Even the lowest-paid woman could do the 'Grand Tour of Europe', she noted. 'Today the typist is putting the lid on her machine and booking a passage to London.'

The title of her first column was pithy and to the point: 'Bargains in Travel'. 'Travelling inexpensively, more often than not, gives one a much deeper insight into and appreciation of foreign countries than deluxe travel can give,' Weekes told her readers airily.

Later in life, after all the bike riding and mountain climbing, Weekes would come to enjoy first-class accommodation, limousines, and an early flight on the first Concorde. However, none of her published travel writing would celebrate or recommend luxury for its own sake.

On the other hand, the cheapest option was not necessarily the best. Weekes advised against paying the minimum rate on a steamship to London, an option that may have meant an inside cabin with no porthole. 'Automatic airshoots are all very fine in theory, but in practice they aren't even a second cousin by marriage to a porthole.'

Weekes' writing developed a tone of gossipy authority, and it was clear she revelled in it. She warned that 'the average person cannot gauge the possible comfort of the ship from a shore inspection or even by looking at the plan of the ship'. In her opinion, it was more important not to be confined to limited deck space 'and to be able to place one's deckchair amidships in rough weather, than it is to have the luxury of switching the light on and off over one's pillow. And yet it is that bedside switch that often determines the prospective voyager.'

Knowing the power of the honorific, she went under the by-line Dr Claire Weekes, yet her informative columns were unpretentious. Should you wish to walk, catch a train, live cheaply, live well, understand history, enjoy art or music, or soak up the local culture, Weekes catered for all tastes.

She started with the basics: how to prepare for a trip, what to wear, how to budget, what to expect — even reviewing third-class train travel, which she heartily endorsed (a side benefit was being able to join in singing folk songs). She offered seasonally adjusted tours through Europe for the uninformed, as well as the classically inclined, finding hotels and cafes as breezily and comprehensively as she compared Renaissance painters or recommended classical music tours.

Although she knew and understood musical history and the geography of Beethoven, Brahms, Schubert, and Mozart, she published under headlines such as: 'Preparation Means Saving of Time and Money En Route', 'Problem of Foreign Languages: English Sufficient in Most European Countries', or 'How to Use That Spare Time before the Ship Sails'.

For the artistically ignorant, she offered both sage advice and a method, and in doing so demonstrated the depth of her own cultural education. 'You just tackle the artists in chronological order. This need only be done in one gallery,' she explained. Start with the Louvre. 'Afterwards no gallery in Europe will present difficulties. A van Eyck beside a Vermeer may not seem anything so extraordinary but put a van Eyck beside other paintings of the

15th century and it opens the eye of the beholder to the heights achieved by this 15th century Flemish painter.'

Only occasionally in this long exercise in writing for newspapers did she veer into the personal. On 6 March 1938, in Weekly Travel Service No. 69, entitled 'Few Days from Paris: Castles of the Loire', she recommended Aurousseau's travel books. There was no mention of their relationship, but it was a blatant plug: 'Marcel Aurousseau, a writer of whom Australia can be justly proud, describes Bourges most satisfyingly in his book "Highway to Spain," which is one of the few good travel books written this century,' she wrote with evident warmth.

Perhaps most subtly personal of all was her report on the controversy over a large sculpture of a female, called *Rima*, by the sculptor Jacob Epstein. A monument to the novelist, naturalist, and ornithologist W.H. Hudson, it sat in a secluded section of Hyde Park. First unveiled in 1925, it was dubbed 'The Hyde Park Atrocity', its offence being twofold. It was a sexually charged sculpture of a woman, arms akimbo, and it stood without the protective cover of classical sculpture, instead harking to themes from non-Western art. The large stone female relief was surrounded by some grotesque birds. In July 1938, Weekes tackled the subject, albeit briefly. Under the heading 'Sunshine in Hyde Park and Kensington Gardens', she wrote:

> The paths now lead straight ahead to the Bird Sanctuary and to Rima, that much discussed statue by Epstein and memorial to WH Hudson. What can be said of Rima? Some say she is beautiful and express their appreciation convincingly; others say she is beautiful because they think it is the right thing to say; others do not think about it at all; and others, perhaps the big, inarticulate majority, think she is so ugly that some of them bring

buckets of tar and bags of feathers to help express their opinion. Poor Rima. Poor Epstein. Poor Hudson. Poor majority.

Weekes might have been writing for the majority, but she was in a minority. She had gone abroad with Elizabeth Coleman and she had returned with her 'Beth'. Weekes would prove on many occasions to be ahead of her time, and this broadside against critics of the Epstein statue hinted at a particularly modern approach to social attitudes, especially in relationship to women.

While Weekes worked every day of the week, Alan and Brian now had busy social lives. Her brothers had carried their London jobs home, and both men lived comfortably, working for multi-national advertising agencies. Advertising paid well for writers, artists, and musicians. Alan eventually became a 'jinglesmith', a job requiring the deft marriage of words and music, with the most memorable ditty he wrote in later years being for Australia's famous breakfast spread, the dark, tarry substance known as Vegemite. 'We're happy little Vegemites, as bright as bright can be, we all enjoy our Vegemite for breakfast lunch and tea', was almost a national anthem, although the appeal of this salty beef-based unguent was often inexplicable to non-Australians.

As her brothers gallivanted on the corporate account, Weekes worked and kept Beth Coleman close. In the '30s and '40s, the two women either stayed at Bellevue Hill with Fan and Ralph, or, less often, travelled to the Upper North Shore to Chatswood to stay with Coleman's family.

While Alan appeared in the social pages for his organising of charity balls, Weekes was mentioned, too, often secondarily to Coleman and her achievements, but also for various public speeches, usually on the subject of travel, now that she was a 'specialist' in the field. The journalists kept up with progress on her guidebook, and the adjective 'brilliant' was occasionally attached to her name. The doctorate lived on.

By April 1939, Weekes' guidebook was almost finished and was due to be published before the end of the year. Queensland was 'the only state which she had not yet covered'. She was pressing ahead, her enthusiasm undiminished by news from abroad. Despite direct experience of the troubles in Germany, she had not anticipated war. If there was one black hole in her unusually good observatory, it was politics.

In March 1938, just as Weekes launched her travel business, Hitler annexed Austria in the Anschluss. Weekes, oblivious to the growing tensions, continued to recommend touring opportunities there. As late as 13 August 1939, she wrote 'Vienna Was Made for Sight-Seeing'. This was followed the next week by 'Music in Vienna: Visiting Beethoven's House'. She also mentioned the Führer in one of her columns, recommending a tour of his house in the south-east corner of the Alps. On Sunday 27 August 1939, her column was headlined 'Lilac Time in the Vienna Woods', and this innocent essay was her last. On 1 September 1939, Hitler invaded Poland, triggering World War II. The only prospective travellers to Europe would be men in uniform.

Weekes' almost-completed guidebook, her weekly column, and her income toppled over simultaneously. Her venture could not have been more poorly timed. The best that could be said was that she gained experience in shaping stories for a wide, general audience. Records from the Women's College Roll at the University of Sydney briefly recorded the moment: 'unable to publish Guide Book on Australia'.

When war was declared, Weekes was still living in the family home, with her parents, at 32 Fairweather Street, Bellevue Hill. Coleman came and went. In 1940, Alan joined the Royal Australian Air Force. Brian joined the army and volunteered for foreign service but remained in Australia, his art skills apparently coming in handy as a designer of material that would help camouflage servicemen and baffle the enemy.[6] Alan's creative muse was unable to be completely boxed in by the war, and there were reports of 'Merry-making Airmen' in a revue called 'Keep 'Em Flying', which was performed in Melbourne.[7]

While war determined her brothers' fates, Weekes was now facing yet another career impasse at the age of 37. Her plans had not been entirely fantastic, had been more than precariously linked to reality, but they showed a capacity for impulse, as well as adventure. Yet Weekes had perseverance. Her nieces remember a judicious woman who kept calm. She was a model of disciplined restraint, in their eyes.

War had its sobering effect, and Weekes was old enough to remember well its predecessor. In 1916, her 28-year-old Uncle Herbert — Fan's brother — had died on the Somme in the Battle of Pozières, in which Aurousseau had also been wounded. As she contemplated her next career move, she must have ruminated on how her own experience fitted what she already understood about such fraught, tragic times. The consequences of war had layers of personal meaning for her, not least among them the inevitability of 'shell shocked' soldiers.

Perhaps with her eye on how her past might service the future, she made another signature leap. In 1941, Weekes enrolled as a mature-age student in the Faculty of Medicine at the University of Sydney. The faculty, even in wartime, was dominated by men by a ratio of six to one. Weekes was given one year's credit for her science doctorate, and, four years later, she graduated as a doctor, just as the soldiers were making their way home.

In *Shell Shock and Its Lessons*, Elliot Smith and Pear identified the importance of the primary physician in treating mental disorders. 'It is an indisputable fact that many modern physicians are apt to concentrate their attention almost exclusively upon the bodily ills of their patients. Yet the majority of doctors, especially those who in general practice get to know their patients intimately, admit readily, even eagerly, that not a small number of the maladies which come under their notice are seriously complicated, if not dominated, by mental factors.'

Weekes did not need telling, and she would certainly 'get to know her patients intimately'. Although she had now returned to a more conventional path, she would find a way of turning it into a unique journey — one that would lead her to her second global reputation.

Chapter 14

THE WORLD AT WAR

Brian and Alan married just as the war broke out, and these new connections in the family would eventually pull both men away from their controlling mother as well as open the door to a set of new strains within a few short years. The women the young men wed came from wealthy families, but that was about all they had in common. Brian married Noel Skarratt, whom he called his 'wild child'; the Skarratts were wealthy and English, and despaired of their daughter marrying a 'socialist'. Alan on the other hand married into the powerful Wentworth family, with guests at his wedding to Joan Wentworth including a knight of the realm, members of the powerful Fairfax newspaper dynasty, and a future prime minister, Billy McMahon.

The latter marriage rang the closing bell on the relationship between Alan and his family. Only Claire would survive the estrangement. Fan's two boys had married above their mother's station, and she was keenly conscious of this. She may have ranked them below their brilliant and compliant sister Claire, but Brian and Alan had stepped out and up, and the mother was intimidated by the in-laws they delivered. Weekes herself had a natural confidence, reinforced by her achievements. She had a touch of her mother's sensitivity to status, but never lacked a sense of her own importance.

After the marriages came the war, and with Maclaren on overseas service, Dulcie moved back into the family home at Bellevue Hill with her two-year-old daughter, Frances. Like her elder sister, Dulcie disliked being alone, and Fan was more than happy to have both of her daughters living with her. Ralph, sidelined for the main part, was banished to the back room near the garage. One excuse for his despatch was that the room doubled as a studio and allowed him space to paint, but Ralph's health was deteriorating, and his hearing was failing. This was a cruel fate for a musician, and Ralph tried to make an income from painting mirrors, just as his father had before him. Weekes graduated to the front parental bedroom, which she shared with Coleman, and Fan took the small back bedroom. A new pecking order was established.

Fan had her own fears. She was convinced the Japanese would target Sydney Harbour, that her family, who lived just above it on a ridge, were at risk of being blown up. 'The house was near the water, near flying boats. She had a thing about the Japanese coming into the harbour, and she was right!' recalls Frances.

As a result, the Weekes family kept on the move over the war years. When Fan had an intimation the enemy was on its way, she led her brood to boarding houses north of the city, and, on one occasion, in 1942, she took them as far as 500 kilometres from Sydney. A few months later, Japanese midget submarines entered Sydney Harbour and blew up a ferry, leading to the loss of over 20 lives.

That evacuation was memorable for one member of the family. For some reason, when Fan whisked them all away to a country station, Ralph was banished instead to a nearby country town, Armidale, where he melted down in misery and rage, his impotence and vulnerability on high beam in a letter to his neighbours Clarrie and Ethel Seccombe back home in Sydney.

> How are you getting on down there, I wish I were with you. I think this is the last place on earth one would want to live in, the heat is something vile, day after day. I don't think I'll be able to stick it much longer. Don't be surprised to see me knocking at your door any night. Mrs W and family are in a large station in the country and I am here on my own, very very lonely. I think they are mad to break up the home.
>
> Where I'm staying is full of women (very common from Newcastle) and children from babies in arms to 12 years old, 18 of them crying and fighting all day. You can picture the good time I'm having ('oh yeah'). I can't strike one card player here, no bridge, no anything, just heat and loneliness. It is impossible to get a good place to stay at; they are all very very bad. I hope you are all well. I think of you every night wishing I were with you …

Amid the toing and froing, Weekes studied medicine and Coleman worked at the Conservatorium and the two women spent as much time together as they could. Coleman was accepted by Fan at the outset, although, as time passed, there were tensions. The relationship with Dulcie was tricky from the beginning. Coleman was competition for her sister's time, attention, and affection.

On the other side of the world, as the war raged, two friends who had been vital to Weekes in her 20s found their own path to marriage — finally anchoring a long, unmoored relationship. Cecily Vance had doggedly pursued Marcel Aurousseau in London for almost a decade to no avail. An opportunity for increased intimacy presented itself after Aurousseau's lodging house was bombed in one of the very early German raids on London in 1940 and he was injured.

Unflustered, Aurousseau carried on with his mapping work despite his injury, 'sleeping in the Royal Geographic Society's building on a stretcher for a fortnight', only seeking medical attention after a period when he could neither walk nor balance and was seeing double. The doctors were baffled, but he was later diagnosed with damage to his ocular nerves.

The problem was fixed by time, which turned out to be on Vance's side as she was given an opportunity to look after him. On 3 April 1941, *The Sydney Morning Herald* reported on a 'recent London wedding. Mrs E Vance of Cremorne has just received a cable from her daughter, Miss Cecily Mary Vance, telling of her marriage to Mr Marcel Aurousseau in London recently'.

Aurousseau acknowledged that it took him time to appreciate Vance's potential as a wife. 'I don't know how it came about, but I managed to get myself married to an Australian friend who was in London at the time. She herself said it took a major war to bring me to this point.'[1] It was an enduring and successful union, lasting until Aurousseau's death in 1983 at the age of 95. The couple maintained a long and strong friendship with Weekes, suggesting she had not been so martyred after all.

They married the year Weekes enrolled in medicine, and her medical studies absorbed the remaining four years of the war, the last twelve months of which were a truly testing time. She was forced, after a period of ill health, and soon after her final exams, to undergo a hysterectomy. This was surgery requiring significant recuperation time, and it left her weary and lacking energy. She returned to work far too soon, yet later expressed pride in how she had managed both her health and her internship at the Rachel Forster Hospital, drawn to the all-female medical staff and its mission to improve the health of women and children.

Chapter 15

DR WEEKES, REDUX

Weekes graduated as a doctor of medicine in March 1945, at the age of 42. As usual, this new achievement by Weekes, now a 'doctor' for the second time, made the newspapers. One carried a photo of her under the headline: 'Women change-over studies ... deny they are fickle'. 'Why is it,' a journalist writing for *The Sydney Morning Herald* wanted to know, 'that women who study for years and attain University degrees or other diplomas switch suddenly to work of quite a different nature.'[1]

While the writer was impressed with Weekes' 'brilliant career' and listed all of her academic achievements, Weekes and the other three women who were interviewed had to deny 'that they were fickle, unstable, or did not know their own minds'. The story concluded that 'women, particularly those who did not marry, gravitated naturally towards the jobs which offered the most personal element'.

Weekes' Faculty of Medicine yearbook came roughly to the same conclusion. Weekes was good with people. It recorded that 'if the gratitude of patients for sympathy and understanding is an index of success in medicine, Claire's success is assured'.

By the time she donned academic robes to receive her medical degree, she was already working at Rachel Forster, in Redfern. Named for a governor-general's wife, a supporter of the suffragette Emmeline Pankhurst, Rachel Forster was a well-established institution when Weekes arrived. In 1941, it serviced over 126 inpatient beds, treated hundreds of outpatients daily, and became a training school for general nurses and a Sydney University Teaching Hospital for medical and surgical undergraduate students.

Weekes' internship was demanding, even for someone with her stamina. She worked three or four days at a time with little if any sleep. It was a system reliant on youthful vigour, and most of the other interns were two decades younger. Professional life for Weekes was now set by predictable compass points, although there would be little respite from work and she was uninclined to set limits, but, in 1947, there were upheavals in her wider family.

On 7 January, her brother Brian was granted a divorce from Noel on the grounds of desertion and noncompliance. Their daughter, Penny, was a toddler and was juggled between her grandparents.

Later that year, the 68-year-old Ralph died. His last few years had not been easy, as his physical and mental health deteriorated. Dulcie's husband, Maclaren, fumed years later to his daughter Frances that he thought Fan treated Ralph very poorly, that he seemed an outsider in his own home.

The household now shrank to Fan and Weekes, although Coleman spent time there. Maclaren had returned from the war, and he and Dulcie were living on the other side of the harbour. All the household chores were done by Fan, and her working daughter was exempt from domestic demands. Weekes' contribution was of the traditional masculine currency for that era. She owned her own car, painted rooms, and earned an income. There was an expectation she would always look after her mother.

By the late 1940s, Weekes had completed her internship at Rachel Forster and opened her own general practice in Sydney's beachside suburb of Bondi, not far from home in Bellevue Hill. She continued her association with the Rachel Forster Hospital until her retirement.

According to her extended family, Weekes was a gifted diagnostician, possibly underpinned by her fastidious attention to what was physical illness and what was not. Sir Grafton Elliot Smith, her earlier mentor, had noted with disapproval in 1917 the absence of understanding of mental illness among general practitioners. It 'may seem remarkable that the medical profession as a whole should take so little interest in, and know so little of psychology,' he observed.

Weekes did not make this mistake; her empathy meter was on the highest setting. She rankled over a lifetime about the incompetent, insensitive medical treatment that had extended her own suffering in her 20s. She knew the power of the doctor, for better or worse. Her nervously ill patients now had the advantage of a doctor who understood both their physical and mental ills and could untangle them.

In the Sydney suburbs, Weekes, with her antenna for anxiety, found suffering in all its varied manifestations. The empathy identified by her medical colleagues now found a river of need and she jumped right in. Her patients 'taught her', she later said. She 'heard everything' and saw the different ways — mental and physical — in which anxiety clothed itself.

There were those homebound with the condition later known as agoraphobia. Then there were the phobics, the obsessives, those tortured by a particular problem, and the just plain miserable. Determined not to repeat the medical mistakes she blamed for her own suffering, she explicitly treated 'nerves' when she found them. Anxiety, however, was not a condition amenable to the 15-minute consultation, and so began the habit of a lifetime whereby these patients were given time and attention above and beyond conventional expectations. It was also the beginning of Weekes' closely watched empirical studies of what she deemed 'nervous illness'. Later, she would tell British psychology professor Roger Baker that she was especially interested in 'the effect of any accompanying nervous illness on physical disease'.[2]

Her growing expertise did not enrich her, as her gift of time was literally that. While her consultations were infinitely elastic, her fee was fixed. The reward for her medical model, based as it was on unlimited time and patience, was not money but validation. For a long time, her patients' gratitude was her only repayment. One day it would not be quite enough, but money would not be the problem.

Two decades as a doctor extended her understanding of those 'tricks' of the nerves, and she didn't need to leave home to study the phenomenon. Dulcie was Exhibit A, Maclaren drank too much, and Brian's mood swings were notorious, while his ex-wife, Noel, who kept in contact, was seriously troubled.

From the outset of her career as a doctor, Weekes made home visits, driving herself to attend to women locked away in suburbs on home duties. Sometimes, she took one of her nieces, who would wait outside in her beloved Vauxhall. The extended family of the '50s was atomised by the ubiquitous car. Women were actively discouraged from working, and their husbands ruled either benignly or otherwise — and some carried into the home the stress of the war years. The lessons of World War I had not been learned. After World War II, men were expected to just get on with it, as were women.

Society, as always, was in transition. Divorce, barely thinkable in the previous generation, was more common, but the law required a blame game, which was then played out in the excruciating glare of the public eye. Court battles were a great source of lurid news-paper articles.

Weekes noted how lack of occupation affected some women, locked into domestic life. It was made worse with a difficult husband. She also knew there were many men who genuinely helped their suffering wives, but she was familiar with those who either wouldn't or couldn't.

Anxiety was not gender-specific — and she made the point often — but men had work to keep their minds occupied, and they often self-medicated with alcohol, in public bars that remained a male preserve, while women were underemployed and could face a frustrated or hostile partner at the end of the day.

She saw how little understanding was available for her anxious patients. 'As I've always said, nervous illness is a very lonely busi-ness, because most people cannot expect support from their family. If they get it, it's just fantastic. But as a rule, many nervously ill people get no support from their family.'

Weekes hated conflict and tended to indulge difficult men. To lessen their impatience with their broken wives, she harnessed her powers of insincerity, telling them they were the 'wise ones in the family'. She empathised, telling them that 'living with [a woman's] nervous system seems like living with live wires'.

Weekes was privy to confessions of alarming fantasies and phobias, from the pilot afraid of flying, the mother afraid of harming her child, the spouse fearing they hated their partner, and many more private imaginings. Then there was guilt and shame, about events real or imagined, that bombed the brain. Finally, there were those shredded by some seemingly unmanageable problem or relationship.

Those years of closely watching humans eventually deliv-ered a better return than the time spent observing lizards. When her books on nervous illness became bestsellers, the American psychiatrist Dr Manuel Zane identified Weekes' 'careful, open-minded, accurate observations of a constantly changing phenomenon, phobic behaviour'.[3]

Zane understood the effort, reflected in the success of her books, that Weekes had put in to 'gaining access to the patient's unique, private experiences in the phobic and therapeutic situations. This objective information, available only to an interested, inquiring human being is indispensable for the development of a scientific understanding of disturbed behaviour and for effectively treating fears and phobias.'

Like Professor Harrison before him, Zane lamented that the sort of 'open-minded, highly personal observation approach' Weekes practised was being 'seriously neglected'. He quoted the Nobel Prize winner in Physiology or Medicine in 1973, Nikolaas Tinbergen, who warned against the trend to look down on the 'basic scientific method' of observation and instead favour 'the glamour of apparatus and prestige of tests' and 'the temptation to turn to drugs'.[4]

In 1955, at the age of 52, Weekes aimed for the next rung on the medical ladder by sitting the examination for membership of the Royal Australasian College of Physicians. Those who passed became members of the RACP and were entitled to call themselves 'physician'.

Established in the 1930s, the RACP was modelled on its British equivalent, which aimed to increase the prestige of doctors, by anointing a higher cadre. The move presaged medical specialties, and, along with the goal of enhancing the status of the medical profession, there were practical objectives, such as promoting research and ethical practices.

Having studied and sat for postgraduate exams, the newly qualified physician tended to then specialise, although some, like Weekes, chose to be general physicians, meaning they were high-level diagnosticians and problem solvers. The category still exists today, although they are more elusive in an era of specialisation.

Having qualified as a physician, Weekes moved into rooms in Sydney's Macquarie Street, a locational synonym for specialist treatment before Sydney's suburban sprawl made such centralisation impractical.

Weekes had not forgotten the war, and she offered her services as a consultant to the Red Cross, where she ran into difficult cases. One was a chemical-weapons scientist, convinced his problems stemmed from nerve gas he had been exposed to while working for the government in Australia. Weekes concurred, diagnosing in July 1960 that his memory loss could be attributed to this exposure, a controversial finding given that governments were highly secretive about the effect of these toxins and only decades later acknowledged the damage.

Once settled in Macquarie Street as a diagnostician, other doctors referred their 'difficult' patients to her, according to Weekes' niece Tita. She had word-of-mouth operating in her favour. What wasn't passed on from Macquarie Street, came from 'Main Street', as her patients referred others.

Her family saw evidence of her diagnostic skills, and, sometime in the late 1950s, Frances introduced Weekes to her mother-in-law, who apparently had Addison's disease. Just by looking at her, Weekes correctly identified that she had been wrongly diagnosed. 'I don't think you have Addison's disease and I think you should get off cortisone straightaway,' her niece remembers her advising her mother-in-law.

Weekes may have had more than one reason to understand the way Addison's disease presented as it was a rare autoimmune condition that attacked the adrenal glands. More importantly, it was the disease, named after Thomas Addison's 1855 discovery, that 'inaugurated the study of the diseases of the "ductless glands"' Weekes had studied under Elliot Smith years before in London.

As her reputation grew, Weekes attributed her success to the years of training prior to medicine as a research scientist, which, she said 'helped me very much to analyse what was happening to a patient and to see the simplicity that lay behind the whole pattern of their nervous suffering'.[5] Science trained her 'to search for the trunk of the tree', as she put it, rather than being distracted by the leaves on the branches. 'I was able to pick, I thought, the most important part of an illness and people's reactions.'

Being a general physician, she saw more than her share of anxious patients: those with a racing heart that challenged the cardiologist, the stomach problems that baffled the gastroenterologist, the eye problems with no explanation, the lump in the throat that could be felt but not seen, among many other 'tricks of the nerves'.

She began to question psychiatric treatment. 'Psychoanalysis often called for a search for possible subconscious causes, a search which could demand weeks, months, even years. Not only were anxious apprehensive people sometimes warned of the necessity of such long searching, the encouraging word "cure" was rarely used. It was even purposely avoided.'

People began seeking her out for urgent relief, from attacks of panic, rapidly beating hearts, weakness, fatigue, trembling, a feeling of difficulty in swallowing solid food, and so on. 'Can you imagine such people's bewilderment and despair on being told of the possibility of lengthy investigation for a hidden cause?'[6]

Weekes had qualified as a physician, but there remained one higher rung on the medical ladder. The RACP had an elite group of 'fellows', a jealously guarded distinction which was the gift of those who had mysteriously been already chosen. In later years the appointment of 'fellows' would become more transparent, as the 'members' objected to this unaccountable and opaque club. However, before this tiny revolution, Weekes was nominated as a 'fellow', an honour and recognition that gave her much satisfaction.

While Weekes was keen to prove herself an exemplar of medical professionalism, her approach had uncommon and unorthodox elements. First, there was the amount of time she gave her patients, going far beyond standard practice. Her phone never stopped ringing; her work was never done, and flowed from the surgery into her home, where her mother and Coleman ensured she was given all the time she needed with her patients. The two women who loved her saw the results she was getting. They thought she was brilliant, and enabled her work.

The rest of the Weekes family, meanwhile, seemed settled enough, but only at first glance. By 1949, Brian had married his second wife, Esther, with whom he had two children, Timothy and Barbara. Esther was the opposite of a wild child. Compliant and loving, she was loved back as Brian's tender letters to her over the years would demonstrate. Yet Brian's genuine affection for his second wife did not inhibit his savage tongue, and he shamelessly humiliated her in public over the years.

Of all the siblings, it was Dulcie who played the largest part in Weekes' life, for better or worse. Weekes dearly loved her younger sister, despite their many differences. Dulcie stepped into the role of housekeeper, which Weekes willingly ceded to her. She led a quiet life but enjoyed the domestic arts that bored her sister, such as cooking, knitting, and dressmaking, and had the Weekes talent for music. A skilled pianist, Dulcie composed her own songs, including one about bossy Fan, called 'What Will We Do with Grandma?' with lines like 'she's 82 and just like new' and 'she tells our friends what they ought to do, and if we complain she tells us too'. Soft-hearted and fragile, Dulcie loved a laugh and a chat, like most of the Weekeses. She fell readily into second place.

Weekes' relationship with Dulcie's husband had started out well, so much so that Weekes had moved in with them on her return from Europe and when they were first married. At the time, the Maclarens lived close to the city at Darling Point.

The harmony did not last long. Maclaren was a fascinating handful. He had a journalist's gift for droll communication, as well as the occupational inclination to drink. Postwar, however, he became an alcoholic. When he finally reformed in his last few years, he told his daughter that, like W.C. Fields, he would have 'liked to live it all over again, without the booze'.

Dulcie and Maclaren eventually moved quite a distance away from the Weekes-family home at Bellevue Hill to Wahroonga, a leafy suburb across the harbour. It was close to an expensive private girls' school, Abbotsleigh. Weekes would one day pay the school fees there for Frances. All of Dulcie's girls — Frances, Lili, and Tita — would be the beneficiaries of her passion for education, and Weekes met the bills for all three of her nieces, at various private schools.

Whatever Weekes did for his family was significant enough to inspire Maclaren to bestow on his sister-in-law a very personal gift — the watch he had been given by his family on his 21st birthday. As it came from his mother's family firm, the Muir and Nicol jewellers in Sauchiehall Street, Glasgow, this was no idle gesture.

The emotional connection was soon savagely reversed with bitterness that lasted a lifetime on all sides. Maclaren's love of women took a particularly torrid turn when, in the early 1950s, the dashing Scotsman and father of three young girls had an affair. This was bad enough, but worse was that his lover was Dulcie's attractive cousin, Josephine Ingleton, nee Weekes.

At some stage, Dulcie got wind of the affair and confided in her sister. The two women decided to bust him, with typically fierce encouragement from Fan. It was a risky, distasteful scheme, but it was in keeping with the times. First shame, then blame, and then gain an advantage in the divorce that followed, under laws that demanded gritty evidence of marital breakdown. Dulcie, however, was uninterested in that excoriating legal game. Divorce was the very last thing on her mind. All she wanted was to shame her husband into returning home, but Maclaren refused to follow her script.

He wanted a divorce, but Dulcie refused. However, she found herself captive to the legal proceedings launched by the other aggrieved party in the tragic circus, Geoffrey Ingleton, Josephine's 45-year-old husband. The ensuing court battle gave Weekes and Dulcie a starring role in the dramatic exposé of Maclaren's infidelity. On 27 September, *Truth* carried the headline: 'Newsman Nabbed in Nude with Spouse of a Sailor'.[7]

Weekes, usually described as a 'brilliant doctor', was recast in a seedy soap opera, lurking on the outskirts of a bedroom. Dulcie was called to give evidence in the court case she had never wanted. Sensational copy was easily obtained from the divorce courts, and the tabloid *Truth* made the most of it. Maclaren would have known what to expect as it was edited by his old boss, Ezra Norton.

> All was quiet in a darkened bedroom at a house in Woolwich Rd, Hunters Hill on the night of April 8 when two women called. The callers, Mrs Dulcie Maclaren and her sister, Dr Claire Weekes, opened the door and switched on the light. A nude man sprang from the bed at the same time accidentally pulling off the bed clothes from the nude woman. And all the nude woman did was to cover her face with her hands.

Truth added that 'Mrs Ingleton is now 40 years old, and still attractive.'

Under the subheading 'Saw Enough' was Dulcie's story of the evening:

> When Maclaren jumped out of bed, she said, he threw the bed clothes aside, and the visitors saw Mrs Ingleton, also in the nude. She covered her face with her hands and left her body uncovered, said Mrs Maclaren.
>
> Mrs Maclaren said she told the pair: 'I thought this was what I would find.' Mrs Ingleton replied, according to Mrs Maclaren: 'Oh, everybody knows.' Mrs Ingleton then donned Maclaren's dressing gown while Maclaren procured another to hide his nakedness. Dr Weekes still stood outside the door. Mrs Maclaren invited her in. 'I don't want to come in,' she replied. 'I have seen enough.'

Truth fluffed out the story with titillating detail and occasional commentary, spreading the misery widely. Josephine was described as 'a member of one of Sydney's best-known sporting families', and her brother's political ambitions were identified. She had married Geoffrey at the age of 21.

> While the young Mrs Ingleton brought beauty to the marriage, her husband brought talent. Ingleton is a man of considerable ability. He has written two books, he is an authority on photography, and he is an artist with a flair for high-class etching work.

The newspaper did not fail to miss the scandalising detail: 'Mrs Maclaren, incidentally, is a cousin of Mrs Ingleton. Husband Muir came into journalism after serving in World War II.'

The story included a piece of contested evidence that fore-shadowed further tragedy. Josephine claimed to have cancer, but her husband ascribed her neglect of the family to the affair rather than illness and accused her of misleading him as well as a doctor. The Ingleton divorce was granted.[8]

It was a sordid mess. Dulcie made a last effort to wrestle her husband back before the court case and at one point thought she had succeeded. Optimistically, Weekes packed Dulcie and the three girls into her Vauxhall, and, accompanied by Coleman, they headed from Bellevue Hill to Wahroonga to move the family back in, so they thought, with Maclaren. Instead it was a debacle. Maclaren arrived at the door in an elegant dressing gown and tried to block entry to his sobbing, beseeching wife. The teenage Frances, and the secondborn, Lili, ducked under his blocking arm into the corridor. Eventually, the Vauxhall was turned around, and Weekes drove her distraught sister and the three girls back to Bellevue Hill.

Weekes now had a ready-made family, and, if her life was disrupted, Dulcie's was smashed. Her three children suffered from the family breakdown and their mother's despair. The responsibility for Dulcie fell heavily on Weekes. Fan, Weekes, Coleman, Dulcie, and the three girls were now tied together, and the bond would sometimes rub unkindly. At some stage, Maclaren's gold fob watch, an intimate gift from an earlier time, was returned to him, on his demand. Dr Weekes was now in charge.

Chapter 16

THE HOUSE OF WOMEN

It did not occur to Weekes that her younger sister, with three young children, should do anything other than return home to live with them. A broken home inevitably meant broken finances, but Weekes' income could be stretched to compensate. The problem, however, was not just money. Weekes worked long hours as a GP, and Fan was in her 70s, with health problems following a series of difficult bowel operations. Weekes had no fear of work but house-keeping was for someone else.

As it turned out, someone else was available. Coleman had been moving between Bellevue Hill and Chatswood for the last decade, and, in 1953, she moved in with Weekes permanently. A lifetime of service to Weekes could be measured from the day Coleman left her own mother in Chatswood to help manage the chaotic household across the Harbour Bridge. Weekes was 40 years old and Coleman was 44. They lived together for the rest of their lives.

As a renowned pianist, Coleman was familiar with the spotlight, yet within the Weekes firmament she was a shadowy, little-known presence. The Weekes were mostly strong-minded individuals happy to sit centre stage, while Coleman had a natural reserve.

In the early years, Dulcie was consumed with grief and rage, and only a wretched connection through the courts remained with her ex-husband as she fought him over maintenance. She remained implacably opposed to granting him a divorce, and so Josephine eventually changed her name to Maclaren by deed poll.

While Muir Maclaren made occasional contributions, it fell to Weekes to provide continuity of financial, as well as emotional, support for the family. Weekes was determined to send her three nieces to private schools, and was willing to pay the fees, and so began a tide of financial dependence, and interdependence. This was a wave of responsibility that would take Weekes on an uncomfortable ride from time to time, particularly in her later years. Money solved problems but bred them as well.

For Maclaren, tragedy followed swiftly, for despite her ex-husband's doubts, Josephine did have lung cancer, and she died in 1957. The bitter feud between Dulcie and her former husband raged on, and no tourniquet would ever stem the bad blood.

Maclaren was a popular character in the eastern suburbs. As a journalist, he could spin a yarn. He was a passionate golfer, loved a drink, and had a wide circle of acquaintances. His views on his former sister-in-law were not kept to himself, and so many Sydney professionals — doctors, lawyers, and his great friend, a judge — were to conclude, based on their conversations with Maclaren, that Dr Claire Weekes was a damned difficult woman.

A battle royal was played out by the two feuding parents, often in front of their children. Second to the suffering of Dulcie came the misery of Frances, whose grief was reinforced by public scenes and the unanchored behaviour of her self-obsessed parents. Lili and Tita were under ten years of age, but Frances, aged 15 when Muir left, was devastated. She had lost the father she adored and as the eldest was especially exposed to the disturbing fights between her parents, and struggled over the next decades to cope with the fiery divided loyalties their estrangement ignited. She married early and her first child was born before she turned 21.

Dulcie's unravelling further underlined her older sister's pre-eminence, and the pecking order. Frances feels her mother 'suffered greatly by being the youngest and in the shadow of Aunty Claire and all her brilliance'. Even Dulcie's youngest daughter, Tita, then only seven years old, remembers her mother as 'distraught'. Fan, with her suite of health problems, occasionally snapped, and, on one occasion, brought out the strap and hit Lili for some misdeed until she was covered with welts. She was still crying when Weekes came home from work, and Lili remembers her aunt's fury with Fan.

Although Weekes had been willing to flirt with all sorts of career experiments, which may have suggested an unconventional approach to life, the opposite was true. If anything, she was overly focused, took herself very seriously, strove to stay calm, and had a strong sense of duty, as generations of Weekeses would discover.

Amid the domestic commotion, Weekes' commitments were growing rather than shrinking. She had a clear view of her new responsibilities. 'When the girls' father deserted them, I took over his role,' she later told her secretary Pat Ryder. She reserved time, and money, for Dulcie's daughters. Tita, the youngest and the favourite, remembers that 'even after she had worked all day at Bondi, in surgery, she would come home and read to me. No one ever read to me, so Aunty would read me *Heidi* and I can't tell you how much I looked forward to that. And she was exhausted.'

Lili's recollections are also of an aunt who was 'like a mother'. When her own mother was overwhelmed, it was Weekes to whom Lili turned. 'I used to go to Aunty with any problems at school, and she would help me with schoolwork. She was always there. I just absolutely idolised her.' According to Lili, her aunt regularly counselled calm. 'Don't get excited, and be prepared for disappointment,' she would say to them. 'She always prepared us for disappointment,' Lili says.

With all the comings and goings in Bellevue Hill, it was a tight squeeze. There were three bedrooms at the front and one out the back behind the garage, but even with Weekes and Coleman sharing and the three girls doing the same, it was crowded. Fan imposed on the growing girls her code of conduct. As teenagers they were instructed to never have sex, over and over again. Frances listened with barely one ear and was keen to go out with boys. She remembers having a 'canoodle' on the front porch with a young man one night about 11 o'clock, only to enter the house and find her aunt painting the dining room after a full day's work treating patients.

Coleman struggled for a place in this family that was not her own. Her position was made more difficult by the muted rivalry she faced from Fan and Dulcie. After a couple of years living with a distraught Dulcie and three school-age children, it was obvious that new accommodation was needed — a home to contain them all while corralling the physical and emotional overflow. Weekes wanted some respite from her extended family, and Coleman's ambiguous status needed to be addressed.

Weekes decided to find a larger house for them all so she could continue to support Dulcie and the girls, but at a manageable distance. She needed to keep the family apart as well as together. North of the harbour, she identified a large Federation house, which they turned into two separate apartments. The war had introduced the family to the far side of the Harbour Bridge, which had some of the loveliest water views in topographically blessed Sydney.

On the North Shore, pretty coves were ushered into sight from an undulating landscape, with endlessly varied views through to the expansive harbour. It was a tranquil forested foreshore within spitting distance of the city. Brian's wartime experience working for the army on camouflage at Georges Head, set in the middle of the most beautiful stretch of coastline on the Lower North Shore, sealed his affection for the area, and he may have aroused his sister's interest.

There was also another reason to move north. In 1956, Weekes' close friends Marcel and Cecily Aurousseau returned to Sydney from London to settle into the family home that Marcel had inherited at Balgowlah, also on the north side. Marcel, now 65 years old and retired, had a huge project underway that would keep him busy for almost two decades: the translation of the hundreds of letters of the German explorer Ludwig Leichhardt.

The friendship between Weekes, Cecily, and Marcel had been maintained, despite the separation London and the war had imposed. That year, Marcel turned down the same honour that Weekes herself would accept 30 years later — an MBE. His work as a geographer had made him an invaluable source of information for Allied forces during World War II, given his contribution to military geographical dictionaries.

There was another side to his modesty. Marcel was that rare breed of Australian, an intellectual, and he had little regard for the opinion of his fellow countrymen. He had only been back a year when he wrote that 'thinking is the hardest work one can offer to many Australians who seem to have no sense of its pleasures'.

Cecily and Weekes more than met his high bar, and, although it took him some time to appreciate Cecily's potential as a spouse, he concluded as an elderly man that 'the last 35 years of my life have been the best period of it and that is very largely due to my wife'.[1]

No one in the family doubted what Coleman meant to Weekes. Their deep relationship rattled Dulcie, who resented Coleman's primacy with her sister. Weekes loved Dulcie, but she had chosen Coleman as her life partner. It was a threesome that needed a separating door. This was exactly what they got when they bought a huge, 18-room Federation home at 37 Milson Road, Cremorne.

Frances rued the destruction of some of the original features of a house that could have been heritage-listed were it not for her aunt's modernising of the upstairs apartment. Yet there was a logic to some of the losses. The beautiful big cedar staircase that linked upstairs to downstairs immediately disappeared, although the old fireplaces were kept. Now there were two separate dwellings, and Dulcie and the three girls were sealed downstairs. This arrangement gave Weekes and Coleman some space, but there was no escaping Fan, who moved in with them upstairs. The property was held in a three-way title, equally apportioned between Weekes, Coleman, and Dulcie, which suggested some court actions against Maclaren had had a monetary outcome.

The upstairs half was level with the road and had easy, flat access via an ugly concrete ramp from an old unused tennis court, where cars could be parked. One particularly appealing asset was a generous front verandah, which offered glorious views of Sydney Harbour. Walking around this deck was about as close to outdoor activity as Weekes got for the rest of her life, apart from the occasional game of golf. Her early days of trekking for weeks on end, scrambling up and down mountains, and bike riding in Scandinavian countries were behind her.

No one remembers seeing her choose to go for a walk, or even a swim, although in one of her last books she observed that 'many nervously ill people do not lead active lives during their illness and suffer from lack of exercise — muscles become flabby and legs tire so easily that sitting or lying, instead of walking, is a constant temptation'.[2]

As evidence of a new order, Coleman was given the large front bedroom, with a view over the harbour. By comparison, Weekes' room was spare, with just a single bed against the window, which did not enjoy harbour views. Fan slept in a bedroom off the kitchen. There was an armchair judiciously placed to enjoy the view in the large living room. This was for Weekes, and became known as the 'throne'.

Weekes was an occasional collector in her travels, but, at home, she valued comfort, and convenience. She had picked up a Persian rug and she was passionate about stationery — favouring blue — but, apart from a couple of her brother Brian's paintings and a print of a Vermeer interior that conjured up domestic peace, her walls in Cremorne were mostly unadorned. There were venetian blinds on the window, a contemporary suburban staple offering light while preserving privacy. She was uninterested in fashion. Tita called her the typical 'mustard mix-n-match' dresser. She was neat, but 'like a country woman, she adopted a comfy, easy code of dress, hated the hairdressers, and had a total lack of vanity about her appearance'.

Music was different. Weekes valued a quality sound system and was prepared to pay heavily for it, investing in the latest on offer in an ongoing rivalry with her brother Brian. Listening to music together was a large part of their lives, and her great-nephew Adam still had her Nakamichi stereo 15 years after she died. He remembers where she bought it and how much she paid — '$2,500 or something ridiculously expensive'.

The move consolidated Weekes' position as head of the family. For a lot of the time she was there, Fan was unwell, Dulcie was in mental torment, and her spirited nieces needed attention, particularly as the sedate '50s unfolded into the sexy '60s. Weekes was a financial and emotional provider, but there were limits to the latter in what was often a chaotic and troubled situation.

They were one big family, but there was now, literally, a gate. The entrance to the top floor — and to Aunty Claire — was through a barn door, over which Coleman had hegemony. She could open the top and keep the bottom locked, thereby keeping members of the family at bay, telling them Weekes was working or sleeping in the pattern established by Fan. This arrangement perfectly suited Weekes, who loathed conflict. At Cremorne, Coleman was the temple dog, and Weekes the temple.

Weekes' own passport to independence had been education and she not only paid her nieces' school fees but bought them books and encouraged them. None would be scholars, but all remember her efforts. Dulcie, without a job, or higher education, had her own way of fighting back. At a school concert one day, she was provoked by what she described to her daughters as the 'posh' voice of the mother sitting next to her who had asked her how many children she had. 'Six,' said Dulcie. 'Three legitimate and three illegitimate.'

Yet her eldest sister had her own version of posh. *That* voice, one of her nieces would say. Vowels became more rounded and consonants clipped when Weekes was in England. She carried the authority of the medical professional she was, and her opinions were delivered as well as held.

While Weekes was a second mother to Frances, Lili, and Tita, she also kept an eye on Brian's daughter Penny, and was bothered by the teenager's unsettled life, warning her brother that constant changes to her schooling were disruptive and would limit her academic progress. Over the years, Weekes had recognised Penny's academic promise and actively encouraged her, noticing how little support for her ambitions she got from her father. Penny showed a youthful interest in medicine, and Weekes pressed her to consider attending her own school, Sydney Girls High, and was particularly delighted when Penny matriculated and successfully qualified for medicine. This was possibly the high point of a relationship that would become increasingly complicated for both.

The four nieces she was closest to all came from broken homes, and Weekes made efforts to compensate. She had no need to do the same for Brian's second family as his two children, Barbara and Tim, lived as stable a domestic life as could be possible with such a volatile father. And there was no demand for Weekes across the harbour, where Alan and Joan lived in comfort.

Dulcie's girls called Coleman 'Aunty', but the implied familiarity was misleading. Coleman lived with the Weekeses for decades but remained always an outsider. She never sought to change this status, nor was invited to, and was remembered mainly for her quiet presence, her cooking, and her exceptional devotion to their aunt. Without Coleman, their aunt 'wouldn't have been able to function'.

Little was known about Coleman's family except the scant information that her father was a journalist, that she had brothers and nieces of her own. Coleman perpetuated her invisibility by giving little away of herself. Her only power was derivative — it came from Weekes. Outsiders who knew her recalled an exceptionally kind and warm individual.

After they relocated to Cremorne, a routine was established. Coleman ran the house upstairs, looking after all the domestic duties; Dulcie was left to her own devices downstairs yet was expected to be on call to care for her mother; and Fan herself would bang on the floor with her cane to round up her youngest daughter. The washing machine also lived downstairs with Dulcie, who took responsibility for the entire establishment. As Weekes worked at her practice and Coleman taught at the Con, much of the heavy load of caring for an ageing woman plagued with serious digestive problems fell to Dulcie, which she accepted as her lot.

The kitchen became a point of contention. Fan liked to cook and so did Coleman. The usually compliant Coleman would often end up 'at loggerheads' with Fan, who could be quick with her temper. According to Tita, 'the kitchen was a war zone with

Aunty Beth, Mum, and Nana trying to deliver perfect dishes. Corned beef, roasts, Irish stew, bread-and-butter pudding, tapioca, rice with sultanas. Real *Commonsense Cookery Book* fare.'

Tita would wander in to the kitchen to hear deep sighs, and see arms raised in defeat and eyebrows staring at the ceiling. 'You could slice the tension with a knife.' The ploy to win Weekes' approval was 'never more evident than in the kitchen'. Anyway, Lili says, 'she didn't like cooking, Aunty Claire, so, well, we did spoil her, there's no question about that.'

Coleman 'had a way of sighing', and she also had a way of signing off. When the upstairs barn door was closed, Lili concluded her aunt 'had had enough, so Aunty Beth has just locked the door'.

Tita, who had some sympathy for Coleman's ambiguous status, describes the unspoken message that hung in the air as 'she should not be here'. She believes Coleman wasn't wanted, at least by Dulcie or Fan, and that this sentiment was communicated to others in the family. No one, however, would gainsay Weekes.

If she wouldn't speak up for herself, Coleman would speak up for Weekes. She would get 'cranky, very cranky' with Dulcie, according to Lili. Dulcie relied heavily on her older sister, and Coleman was infuriated by the regularity with which she would drag any problem with her family upstairs. There were plenty of those. Weekes' keen sense of responsibility for her wider family would deliver uneven rewards over the years. Weekes, Lili says, 'took on everything. She took on her own mother, who was ill, she took on her sister, whose husband had left her, she took on her sister's children, all of us, and she had to work.'

Weekes also insisted on being doctor to them all, as well as counsellor. The most difficult challenge was Dulcie, and Weekes once told Frances that she had 'spent many a night talking your mother out of a nervous breakdown'.

She did more than talk; she also prescribed sedatives. Some

in the family held her responsible for the subsequent fog that descended on Dulcie, although no one doubted the weight of Dulcie's anguish was a heavy burden on her elder sister. And Weekes, who had strong misgivings about antidepressants, regarded sedatives less critically and was tolerant of their use in some circumstances.

Her brother Brian was another family member very happy to turn to Weekes for medical advice. His daughter Barbara recalls the regularity of the visits to their aunt, who conveniently lived in the next suburb. Brian was a troubled man, and often just trouble. His boisterous personality, his gift for storytelling, and his passionate socialist politics had a darker side, which made him highly sensitive and hypercritical of people and confined him to bed when it all got too much.

When the darkness descended, like others in the family, he turned to his elder sister for help. Brother and sister would be in and out of each other's houses over a lifetime, and Weekes tolerated his rocky temperament, although she once complained to Penny about her father: 'I have never had a peaceful weekend with Brian. There always had to be a scene. I was always fond of your mother, Brian would have been impossible to live with.'[3]

Brian resented his sister's success and the material comforts it provided, handily overlooking that the two-storey home had also been purchased by Dulcie and Coleman. He actively discouraged Penny from studying medicine. When she won a place in the faculty, as well as a Commonwealth scholarship, she got no support from him. 'I am not going to spend money on you, so another man gets rich,' she was brutally informed.

Penny's medical studies began promisingly, and she passed first year despite having not studied physics or chemistry at school, but family chaos took its toll. Her father was his usual volatile self, but worse was to come as, in the following year, her mother was committed to a psychiatric hospital for several months. Penny failed second-year medicine by a tiny margin, to her great regret in later life. However, romance intervened, and she married a fellow medical student. In later years, Penny returned to university, attaining an honours and postgraduate degree in psychology.

Despite his jealousy, Brian gave his sister the overt respect that he withheld from other women in his life. They sat in their armchairs in the living room in Cremorne and talked for hours. The socialist Brian had no politics in common with the conservative Weekes, but they discussed science, medicine, and music, and reminisced about their travels in Europe. They mused on philosophy as well, having found common ground as non-believers. Death was a special affront to Weekes as it represented the obliteration of all her learning and mastery of life.

While Brian had conquered alcohol, he was always asking Weekes for some new medication that might solve his problems. Weekes' reputation was later built on giving control back to individuals and freeing them from drug dependence, yet she was permissive with tranquillisers for some relatives, and she wrote in her books that there was a place for occasional sedation. She seemed not to have anticipated that some of her relatives would struggle with addiction. As a non-drinker, and with a disciplined work ethic, Weekes was in no danger personally of succumbing, although Frances noted the tide would (very slowly) go out on the 'medicinal' brandy her aunt kept in her wardrobe.

Later, Weekes argued vigorously against the conventional wisdom that depression was caused by a 'chemical imbalance' in the brain. She aimed at work, if not at home, to hand control back to her patients — from the doctor, psychologist, psychiatrist, and pill — but her burdensome relative's demands were often easier to indulge than resist, and Weekes handed out the sleeping pills that Brian would take when he headed to bed for days, pulling the blinds down on the world and puzzling his family. 'He was a very moody guy and we do really think he had, a touch of, or a lot of ...' His daughter Barbara searches for a word. 'Bipolar,' she concludes.

Not much got past the youthful but observant Barbara. She was gently critical in later years of the ease with which the pills were dispensed. 'I think Dulcie probably got caught up in the cycle of whatever she had been prescribed.'

Then there were Brian's rages against his second wife, Esther. 'That's enough,' Weekes would say ineffectually to Brian as he bullied his wife, publicly, relentlessly.

Chapter 17

THE BIRTH OF A BOOK

Over many years, Weekes established a pattern whereby total strangers with nervous illness were invited to move in — first to Bellevue Hill, then to Cremorne — often for lengthy periods. Here was a vivid example of Weekes' determination to help people recover, and a more closely watched empirical study of nerves would be hard to find.

This was hardly standard professional practice, even at a time when the idea of professional 'boundaries' was not so well established. As it turned out, the idea for this unorthodox 24-hour care was not Weekes' own, but came originally from her mother, Fan.

Weekes told the BBC in an interview in the 1980s, that people 'would come to me from various parts of Australia. Australia is a very big place; they come thousands of miles, from Perth to Sydney and I had some of them staying in my home, perhaps three or four at a time. It was very difficult for them staying in a guesthouse, because they wouldn't know what to do with themselves all day. My mother said: "Why don't we have them stay here?"'

It may have been her idea, yet Fan had little affinity with these 'guests', and she talked about them with her usual tough humour. 'We've got another one of Claire's psychos staying,' she would cheerfully inform other family members.

This boundary blurring between patient and doctor accelerated over the years. People started as patients or readers, and then
Weekes would befriend them. Eventually, a handful became business partners as Weekes preferred the help of people she felt truly
understood her work, in place of more professional arrangements.

Treating anxiety would become a mission. She had always
worked hard and expected a lot of herself but was increasingly
convinced she was offering something available nowhere else.
Weekes later wrote that when she first began to practise medicine,
'Freudian analysis was still the treatment of choice for an anxiety
state, including agoraphobia, and so many people are not only *not*
helped by this, some were actually harmed, and some of them came
to me to be rescued.' This notion that she was 'rescuing' people
was reinforced by the number of individuals who told Weekes she
had 'saved' them.

The troubled individuals who shared her home from time to
time also gave her deep exposure to the different ways in which
anxiety could present. This would give her self-help books their
depth. Her mother's support was critical given her early role as
chief housekeeper. Fan was forced to admit that these guests had
their occasional value, particularly on one occasion, when she
accidentally grabbed a live electrical plug and was at risk of serious
injury. Fan reported afterwards that 'one of Claire's psychos' was
walking around singing to herself and just walked over and turned
off the switch'.

Weekes' patients found an easy place in this bustling, bristling
house of women ranging in ages from eight to 80. The outward
symptoms of anxiety in these individuals presented quite differently, which meant Weekes was getting a broad and deep education
in varied manifestations of nervous distress.

There was a gentle, sweet-natured nun called Sister Carmel,
who was in a deep state of despair. She had led a protected life, and

struggled to travel across the city from her nunnery to be treated by Weekes. She was one of the first to move in with the Weekes family in Bellevue Hill. When Weekes told her nieces that Sister Carmel had never seen a movie, the 16-year-old Frances took her to see *Guys and Dolls*, which she apparently enjoyed. Tita remembers, 'she always knitted dolls' clothes for our dolls. And Aunty got her better. She got her well. She had a bad breakdown. It took quite a while that one, I think.'

Another woman washed her hands every five minutes, according to Lili. A more disturbing patient, who lived for months with them, was a young woman not much older than Weekes' nieces. Her father, a respected professional, had apparently been sexually abusing her. After she recovered, she lived a long life as a successful professional herself.

Tita also recalls the 'CEO of a huge corporation' whose wife had rung Weekes as her husband was so ill he could barely speak or dress himself. 'Part of her treatment,' says Tita, 'was that activity was very helpful, that you needed to do something, anything.' The man wanted to be close to Weekes, and so she put him to work in their garden at Cremorne. 'He didn't garden, he just fiddled,' Tita says. He was outside the house, but he was permitted to go and speak to Weekes on and off all day. 'Eighteen months later, this man who could barely speak — because I used to say hello to him, and he would just look — was back at work, the head of another corporation. You would not recognise him.'

All these patients had been collected either through Weekes' general practice in Bondi Junction or, later, from her surgery in Macquarie Street. The custom did not please all members of her family. Tita notes that her aunt 'bought them home whether we wanted it or not — we didn't have any say!' Success meant more patients, and Weekes never put up a fence to keep the anxious at bay. At home and at work, the telephone rang continually.

Decades later, when the habit persisted, Tita became more irritable still. 'I used to go up to Aunty and say, "*Why* can't you just keep your patients out of the house?"' says Tita fiercely. 'She just said, "Because they need it, darling."'

Yet Tita allowed that her aunt was 'born to give everything that she had in her heart. That's what she did. That's all I know, that this woman gave her life to other people. I mean you'd have to see it to understand it, the degree to which she did this.'

It was hard to imagine many doctors happy to adopt her method with difficult cases, and there were always those. When, many years later, in a question-and-answer session at a hospital, Weekes was asked what could be done about a young person who was unwilling to face what they feared most, her answer revealed the gulf between her practice of medicine and the average doctor.

She told the story of her own efforts with an Australian girl whom a psychiatric hospital had concluded would never recover. 'For a year I'd pick her up every morning and take her on my rounds [as a doctor]. I took her on my rounds every day of the week, practically, and sometimes even at weekends. I gradually had her back in a job as a typist.'

Weekes concluded the young man in question 'was a problem for one particular doctor who will need to be very interested in helping him, and he needs a dedicated doctor who will be prepared to take that boy and try and find out what is actually holding him back, what is actually in his mind, what he's thinking about his illness, and try to get him motivated again.'[1]

Fortunately, these were the very painful exceptions but showed how determined Weekes was to understand nervous illness. The recoveries Weekes saw and the gratitude she received confirmed her belief she was offering something unique. No one, she believed, understood the market for her treatment better than she did. By the end of the 1950s, she assessed the need as so great that her work should be made more broadly available.

The idea for a book came about in a roundabout way. One of Weekes' patients, visiting from Melbourne, asked her to 'write it all down to save you going over it with each of us'.[2] He explained that he found the words in her surgery very buoying, but very hard to hold on to once he had left. Weekes' solution was to record all her consultations and give a copy to each patient. Weekes would often say she was taught by her patients, and now she learned the power of repetition and reinforcement. In order to break an established cycle of response, the tired, stressed mind needed constant reminders to hold on to the words that had been so well received face to face in the surgery.

Sir Grafton Elliot Smith had suggested that a detailed manual needed to be written, and Weekes saw her patients needed it, too. They demonstrated to her how the 'habits of fear' needed to be broken.

The books, based as they were on her words in the surgery, had a 'talking to' quality about them, possibly because they had been dictated originally. Weekes heard repeatedly over the years that her readers felt she was speaking directly to them.

Yet if it sounded easy, the reality was different, and Tita, who suffered from anxiety herself, understands better than anyone how much work Weekes put into getting exactly the right words. When she moved back into Cremorne as a single mother in the 1970s, Tita helped out with the transcribing. In this way, she closely observed the extraordinary commitment her aunt made to honing her message, to keeping it simple and clear. There were ruthless revisions and edits.

'She had a very hard job simplifying her work,' says Tita. 'I typed a lot of her work from a Dictaphone, and I'd type and type and type, and she read it and she might keep one line out of 15 pages or something.'

'These people are sick. It's hard enough for them to read a sentence, let alone a whole book,' Weekes told Tita. By keeping it simple 'she reached a lot of people. She was right: keep it simple — and she did,' says Tita.

Yet there was a mystery. Had someone suggested she write a book? Weekes may have thought of it herself, given she had almost completed a travel guidebook, and this was a guide to mental health.

However, before Weekes had a publisher, she had had a literary agent. Percy Reginald Stephensen was well qualified to assess her skills as a doctor and as a writer. When they first met, he was in a parlous physical and mental condition. This was the start of the pattern. An individual in trouble would find Weekes and recognise her work as offering something unavailable anywhere else, then see its huge potential value. A business proposal would be hatched, and they would go into business together, and it would work for a while, until it didn't.

Born in 1901, Stephensen was in his late 50s when he met Weekes. Temperamentally, they were opposites, although both were big personalities. His biographer, Craig Munro, gave his biography the title *Wild Man of Letters*. The description was apt. A volatile and noisy character, Inky, as he was known to friends and enemies alike (of which there were a surplus in the latter category), had originally been fired by a mission to assert Australia's literary culture against a tide of imports.

The word colourful could not touch the rainbow of controversies and crises that attended his life and vexed career as a passionate Australian publisher, book editor, literary agent, and lifelong political agitator. Educated at Oxford, he published D.H. Lawrence and Norman Lindsay, was immortalised as a 'raucous pornographer' in Aldous Huxley's *Point Counter Point*, flirted with communism, made what author Miles Franklin described as 'a muddled transition from far Left to far Right',[3] and became a leading figure in the Australian fascist movement. He championed Indigenous art while holding fiercely anti-Semitic views and then became fiercely pro-Japan at a politically inconvenient time. In the early 1940s, this last posture earned him imprisonment without trial for the duration of World War II. By the time he met Weekes, impecuniosity had reordered his priorities.

Stephensen's need for money collided, in turn, with another man's need for bestsellers. In 1960, an Angus & Robertson director, a New Zealander called Walter Burns, with an implacably commercial agenda, pushed his way to the top, being appointed managing director of this leading Australian publishing house. As Burns gave the commercial priority over the cultural, he put himself at odds with the beating heart of A&R, represented by George Ferguson (the grandson of the founder) and the company's legendary editor, Beatrice Davis. It was a chaotic time, and Stephensen inserted himself into the vortex, launching a successful charm offensive on Burns, oiling his arrow with promises of making A&R more profitable. Stephensen regularly used the word 'bestseller' in his many communications with the commercially minded Burns.

'With your tremendous buying power, you could make or break almost any English publishing house,' Stephensen cajoled, as he also slyly suggested that Ferguson wasn't quite up to the job.[4] Stephensen's ultimate objective was to run his own local publishing 'subsidiary' of A&R, and, although he failed to achieve this, he managed to persuade Burns that he was just the whirlwind needed to blow out the old and sweep in the new at the company. His pitch was based on the bestsellers Burns demanded, and *Self Help for Your Nerves* was to be one of these.

Stephensen was put in charge of paperback publishing, reporting directly to Burns rather than to the publisher, Ferguson.[5] His elevation would be the briefest renaissance, yet when

Stephensen negotiated a contract with Weekes, he was offering not just his proven editing nous, but real publishing clout at A&R.

How Weekes met him was never discovered, but there were a number of opportunities given their neighbourly proximity, living barely a block apart in Cremorne, and his health. There was also Sydney Harbour, whose dazzling beauty may have been the intermediary as they both made efforts to promote and protect it.

While her first book was in the planning stage, Weekes was appointed secretary of the Cremorne Foreshore Protection League, which was battling a development proposal for a 22-storey building on the beautiful harbour foreshore at the end of her road. Thousands of local property owners signed petitions to the local council, and Stephensen may well have been among them. The local council recorded her success a couple of decades later: 'The Cremorne Foreshore Protection League, led by Dr Claire Weekes, opposed the construction of high-rise in that area because of the threat to views. Campaigns about specific developments were won and lost but, in 1960, Council agreed to consult with "neighbours" affected by flat development before approval was given.'

If Stephensen did not meet her locally, it was possible that he was one of her patients. When he became Weekes' agent, he was in a fragile condition. A lifelong heavy drinker and smoker, he had always inclined towards trouble and stress, and now suffered heart problems, which may have predisposed him to an interest in her somatic approach.

Inevitably, the inflammatory reign of Burns and Stephensen ignited an internal revolt at A&R, led by George Ferguson, which ended their short and brutish regime. After just one year, both men were out of the business, along with their ambitious global paperback plans.[6] It was a mess, and there were after-effects, one of which was that the London office, closed down by Burns, was reopened, as Ferguson persuaded the board that its closure had been a massive miscalculation. It was just as well from Weekes' point of view, as without a London office it would have been harder for her to find a publisher in Britain.

When he left the publishing house, Stephensen held on to his job as Weekes' literary agent. She was already under contract to him, and A&R was publishing her book. However, Stephensen was distracted, engaged as he was in open warfare with the writer Xavier Herbert, who was bitterly outraged at what he felt were Stephensen's overstated claims to editing his seminal work *Capricornia*. Herbert declared in capital letters that 'NOONE EDITED CAPRICORNIA BUT MYSELF' in a letter published in *The Bulletin* magazine. The stress on Stephensen continued to build, and Weekes would become increasingly uncomfortable with their collaboration. Yet she had ceded total control of the relationship from the beginning. An A&R internal memo recorded that in their original contract, dated 5 April 1962, 'we were instructed to pay all earnings to P.R.Stephensen as her agent'.[7]

A&R held Weekes' rights to the British market. That left the United States available for Stephensen, and he promised Weekes a publishing contract in the biggest market in the world. Whatever his deficiencies, Stephensen understood the scale of Weekes' ambition and shared her belief that she was a global talent.

Stephensen was gratifyingly enthusiastic, and confident that she could find an audience in the US. Yet as he strove for a bestseller, Stephensen was under serious pressure on several fronts. He was in debt despite winning a libel settlement against the Melbourne *Herald*, which had published wild claims that he had planned to 'murder national leaders' as part of his political activities years before.[8] Such criminality exceeded even troublemaker Stephensen's wildest ambitions. Still, his views remained extreme.

Sometime in early 1962, Stephensen suffered his first heart attack. At this point, *Self Help for Your Nerves* was well underway and set to be published later that year. Despite the serious threat to his health, Stephensen kept working, determined to drum up international interest in Weekes' book.

Among his international publishing contacts was Oliver Swan, an American literary agent with a reputation as a tireless activist for books he believed in. When he died in 1988, *The New York Times* published an obituary headlined 'Oliver Swan, 83, Literary Agent with Eye for Worthy Unknowns'.[9] As the agent for best-selling author Morris West, Swan had experience of Antipodean publishing triumphs.

On 9 April 1962, Swan wrote from America, expressing his pleasure that Stephensen had 'finally found a home for *Self Help For Your Nerves* ... by Dr Claire Weekes'. Swan was optimistic that there were also prospects in the US. It was an encouraging letter. 'There seems to be a good deal of interest here at the moment on the part of Prentice-Hall, who have been giving it very careful consideration and from whom I hope to have some fairly definite work within the next week or 10 days,' Swan wrote, indicating that the running title for the US edition would be *Beat Those Nerves*. 'Should Prentice-Hall finally decide against making an offer, I agree it would make sense to wait until we have copies of the final Australian edition,' he concluded.

When Stephensen received this letter, he was in a state of high anxiety, hardly helpful given the state of his heart. He was continuing to work but was so unwell his doctor had confided to his wife, Winifred, that Stephensen could die at any time. She was beside herself with worry.[10]

Stephensen was sufficiently agitated that one of his stable of authors, Rex Armitage, took it upon himself to warn his friend and literary agent about the importance of learning to 'relax'. If Armitage was worried about Stephensen, it was serious. This was the author of the self-help book titled *I Beat Both Drink and Dope:*

the authentic autobiography of a drunkard and drug addict who made a complete recovery and *Drunkards Can Be Cured*.

'My Dear Percy,' Armitage wrote, 'You paid me the compliment of telling me I had "a good grip on life", so perhaps you won't mind taking a little well meant advice from me. I am, at 55, in good health despite a "tough" life. And why? Because I am an expert "relaxer". I actually spent some years studying, at the public library, the art of relaxing. I work hard (when I do work), and I relax hard when I relax … in your present state of health, you must for a period, cut yourself off from all worry and unpleasant work. I'm not joking …' He told Stephensen he had 'finally emerged from what was really a more serious illness than you now suffer'.[11]

In this fragile state, Stephensen was in constant contact with Weekes, and, as her agent, he would have intimate knowledge of her method. She could hardly have failed to notice that he suffered from nerves himself. Their relationship deteriorated throughout, and Weekes found him extremely difficult to deal with. Xavier Herbert's rage at what he believed were Stephensen's overblown editing claims gave a clue to the possible trouble. Stephensen had incorrigible self-belief and had opined to his wife that he had saved various writers from themselves. But if Stephensen had tried to control the words of Dr Claire Weekes, he would have met implacable resistance. She had fierce views on the power of the doctor's words to help or harm.

While Stephensen struggled with his health, Weekes was not immune from pressure herself. Though excited about her forthcoming book, she was still a full-time doctor, juggling work, the book, Dulcie, two teenage nieces, and her ill, anxious literary agent. On top of that, there was her ailing mother. Dulcie, who had no job, managed Fan's daily needs, but Weekes looked after the medical side of her mother's care, in the upstairs apartment they shared. Weekes also paid a widow, Mrs Grey, for housekeeping.

On 11 February 1962, Fan died. She was 84, and, although she had been frail and her death was not completely unexpected, it was another distressing disruption in a household that already had its share of grief and dysfunction.

Just to add to the building tensions, Dulcie was again upended: Maclaren had fallen in love with a woman called Jean Phillipson and wanted to marry her. There had been no attenuation of Dulcie's rage and anguish at losing her husband, so she again refused him the divorce he badly wanted. It took over a decade before Dulcie's last remaining power was extinguished by legislation allowing no-fault divorce in the early years of the reforming Whitlam Labor government.

While she could punish Maclaren by denying him a divorce, Dulcie had no way of anaesthetising her own pain, and even Coleman's barn door, separating upstairs from downstairs, could not entirely insulate Weekes from the heat of her sister's despair. In the meantime, Jean Phillipson built a relationship with Dulcie's eldest daughter, Frances, who adored her father's new partner. None of these developments improved Dulcie's state of mind. Frances by now was married with a daughter of her own, but Lili and Tita were in their teens, still living at home.

Amid the turmoil, Weekes' first book was born. Angus & Robertson published *Self Help for Your Nerves* in their 1962 spring list. Her medical status was heavily emphasised on the jacket. Weekes dedicated it, 'To the memory of my indomitable mother.'

Chapter 18

SELF HELP FOR YOUR NERVES

On 10 November 1962, the first review was published in *The Sydney Morning Herald*. It did not start well.

> I must admit I approached Dr Weekes's book with both scepticism and misgiving. The title, to begin with, is mildly irritating; it smacks not only of the 'do-it-your-self' craze which has proved so commercially profitable in recent years, but of the verbose treatises on salesman-ship which strew our bookshops and libraries.
>
> Does not one feel heartsick, too, at the strident emphasis of the book's third sentence? 'THE ADVICE GIVEN HERE,' says Dr Weekes, and the capitals are hers, 'WILL DEFINITELY CURE YOU, IF YOU FOLLOW IT.' Furthermore, on the second page, no fewer than three phrases are italicised for added emphasis. It is not a promising beginning.

The reviewer, Robert Bell, persevered, however, and his initial aversion turned to grudging admiration. 'Read on, I suggest. There is nothing, as President Roosevelt claimed thirty years ago, to fear but fear itself! The book's title turns out to be a completely accurate description of its contents, and the reader will be very speedily impressed by Dr Weekes's obvious professional competence.'

Bell saw value in the book for the general reader, 'even those whose nerves are under control'. He provided a neat synthesis of her explanation of the nervous system and the tricks it could play, and revealed her six-word panacea: *Facing, Accepting, Floating, Letting Time Pass*.

Bell got the idea. You don't fight, but yield. He approved of her dismissal of brisk tough talk such as: 'It all depends on you' and 'Your recovery is in your own hands — it's up to you'. 'A great deal of harm has been done by such advice,' he averred.

In his penultimate paragraph, he acknowledged her medical qualifications as a consulting physician at the Rachel Forster Hospital, and concluded that Weekes had written an 'admirably lucid exposition of the subject. It is serious of purpose and will be of help to those who have vainly sought a cure for nerves.'

Yet the reviewer couldn't quite let go of the idea that Weekes lacked credentials. 'But should her prescription, so persuasively argued, be used by sufferers without at least an initial expert diagnosis and advice?' Bell advised seeking out an experienced psychiatrist to get more individual attention.

Weekes had no way of explaining that, as a senior physician, she had been consulted as an 'expert' by patients who had been referred to her by their doctors for years, nor that the point of her book was to meet the needs unmet by psychiatry. Bell's response was her first introduction to what would become a persistent theme. Individuals who read her books or listened to her audios would be overwhelmed with gratitude, professionals with indifference, or worse.

The press coverage nonetheless started to build favourably. On 18 November 1962, eight days after Bell's review, *The Sydney*

Morning Herald published a full-page article under the headline 'You and Your Nerves. "A Sydney doctor answers the question: what makes a nervous breakdown?"'

Weekes had developed a rapport with her editors in A&R, even though Stephensen had, along with Walter Burns, given the publisher so much grief. Some of the original powers had survived the Burns guillotine, notably the longstanding and respected Beatrice Davis. She was Weekes' in-house editor, and had her own views on Weekes' agent.

Whatever Stephensen's misgivings about 'Anguish & Robberson', there was no local publisher bigger or better to publish Weekes' book. He wanted a bestseller and he got one. A&R had no idea they had a publishing sensation on their hands. They thought 500 copies would cover the first month's demand for *Self Help for Your Nerves*. Five hundred sold in three hours.[1]

It turned out that anxiety was hiding in plain sight. It was in homes, in offices, in executive suites, in hospitals, and far too often in asylums. The sales potential was huge. In 1962, there was nothing else like *Self Help for Your Nerves* on the market. Weekes had written it for that very reason. She was defensive about the genre, given that she was twice a doctor, and a respected researcher. She later explained to Robert DuPont the dilemma she faced when choosing how to best showcase her work.

'Originally, I had to decide whether I would approach sufferers through scientific journals, certainly more dignified for me, having already a bit of a reputation as a scientist (14 years as a research worker with work now being taught in universities worldwide), or whether I would go directly to the people whose need of help was urgent.'[2]

She knew the need was not just urgent, but vast. The question was, however, whether words on a page would carry the same power as they did, face to face, delivered by a doctor in the surgery. For one nervous system to break the isolation of another, a connection had to be made. The challenge was to be 'heard' by readers whom she had never met, and who had never heard of her.

Self Help for Your Nerves was published in hardback in September 1962, just as the inaugural Australian Book Week was held in all Australian capital cities. 'Book publishing in this country has come of age,' declared *The Sydney Morning Herald*.

Weekes' utilitarian title sat alongside some illustrious local writers. There was Douglas Stewart's *Rutherford and Other Poems*, Ivan Southall's *Woomera*, Thea Astley's *The Well Dressed Explorer*, along with *Obscenity, Blasphemy, Sedition* by Peter Coleman. They would all be successful books, but the only one that could be called an international bestseller was *Self Help for Your Nerves*. Fan had predicted the outcome accurately, with typical edge. 'My mother told me I had created a Frankenstein and that patients would be ringing up all hours of the day and night,' said Weekes.[3]

The door at the Weekes household opened almost the moment the book was published — people would just turn up at the house. Weekes became well known, very quickly, according to Tita. 'It was just so exciting, I can't tell you how excited she was.'

The book sold steadily from the beginning, with word of mouth and some strong media support from *The Australian Women's Weekly*. This magazine was a phenomenon. The *Weekly* was purportedly the most successful magazine in the Western world, with one in four Australian families buying it every week.[4] Australia had a relatively small population, but the *Weekly* sold in the millions, thriving on its imperishable offerings on the royal family, husband trouble, celebrities, recipes, and fashion, among other staples. It was a measure of their readers' responses that they regularly reported on Weekes' work.

Woven invisibly into the book was the original thread of Weekes' own experience, yet even unrevealed it enhanced the authenticity that so struck readers, many of whom sensed she had inside knowledge. How could she not, as her descriptions of how they felt were so exact? However, this fact went unacknowledged, and Weekes presented as the doctor she was, reassuringly putting distressing mental disarray into its medical context. She told a story of the nervous system, which was translated popularly as the mind–body connection, and it made her famous.

Her own story lay within the pages, camouflaged. She wrote about a male student whose suffering was ended when a soldier friend explained he was being 'bluffed by his nerves'.[5] Tellingly, in this covert story about her own experience with nerves, she had concluded that the 'student' did not live a life free from stress. 'He has similar feelings from time to time, but he knows that they will pass if he relaxes, accepts and floats past them. He has learned how to live with his nerves.' Weekes' confidence that setbacks should not be feared but embraced as a chance to practise 'acceptance' was based on her own experience.

By her own testimony, it was the 'soldier' who supplied some key ingredients, particularly his advice to 'float past all suggestions of self-pity and fear'. Aurousseau's choice of the word 'float' was collected and used in her six-word treatment plan: *face, accept, float, let time pass*. This word, 'float', and the idea it attempted to communicate, was the most difficult of her four instructions to communicate to patients.

'Face', 'accept', and 'let time pass' were unambiguous and easy to grasp. 'Floating' was trickier, yet overlapped with the idea of non-attachment, common to meditation. In later years, popular exposure to Eastern religions made its meaning a little clearer. Yet Aurousseau's use of the word would have no overtones of Buddhist meditation, and neither would hers. What was later described as a state of 'being in the present, accepting things for what they are, i.e. nonjudgmentally'[6] was the equivalent to her shorthand 'float'.

In her second book, Weekes expanded on what she meant by floating as she said she was often asked about it. 'It means to go with the feelings, offering no tense resistance, just as you would, if floating on calm water, let your body go this way and that with the undulating waves. Let the moment of intense suffering float past you or through you. Do not arrest it or stay baulked by it. Loosen towards it.'[7]

Weekes leveraged her authority as a doctor in the book, understanding that there was more to medicine than scholarship. Bedside manner could make all the difference between success and failure. Her explanation of the nervous system was based on her scholarship, but her approach was unscholarly. To amplify the connection with the reader, she wrote her book in the first person. It was like an extended personal letter. The first chapter was 'The Power Within You', and the opening words described her mission.

> If you are reading this book because you are having a nervous breakdown or because your nerves are 'in a bad way', you are the very person to whom it has been written and I shall therefore talk directly to as if you were sitting beside me ... it will not be difficult for you to read this book: it is about you and your nerves, and for this reason you will read with interest, whereas to read an ordinary book or a newspaper may seem an impossibility, or, should you succeed, may leave you more distressed than when you began.[8]

The right words could calm a nervous system, and Weekes had seen and felt the devastating effect of the wrong ones. If the book reached the reader, it was because her message was 'felt' as well as heard and understood. Her explanations were acceptable in the face of what had been experienced as unacceptable. Often, they were far more than that: a revelation accompanied by huge relief.

Weekes had had years of practice in the surgery to test the words to help her patients. Recording her consultations had allowed her to refine her message and synthesise her explanations. She knew that the nervously ill needed a straightforward and uncomplicated manual to read and reread.

What she was offering was quite at odds with contemporary practice. She was incautious by the standards of the time in asserting recovery was not only possible but inevitable if her advice was followed. Psychiatrists and psychologists favoured professional distance.

As the first reviewer identified, she used capital letters and italics as her loudspeaker: 'THE ADVICE GIVEN HERE WILL DEFINITELY CURE YOU', and, 'however deeply involved you may be in nervous breakdown, it is possible to recover and enjoy life again. I emphasise, *however deeply involved*.' Weekes held out more than hope — she offered certainty. Her reader knew all about doubt.

The medicine went down more easily, as it was wrapped in validation, rather than evaluation, of the reader. Weekes had total confidence in the inevitability of recovery if her advice was followed.

Hope and confidence, however, needed a platform on which to rest, and Weekes provided the medicine and the science. The varied symptoms that seemed so unique to the nervously ill were explained in medical rather than psychological terms. Tricks of nerves manifested in all sorts of alarming ways but could be easily understood for what they were.

Weekes described the many roads to panic, nervous illness, and breakdown, but the journey started in the same place, with fear. It was this primal survival instinct that tuned the nervous system to herald a dissonant orchestra of arousal that could wreak such havoc.

Self Help for Your Nerves was written as a guide. This is the path that took you into the dark, this is how and why you got lost, and here is the path out. The appeal of the book was how easy it was to understand, yet what looked so self-evident was not, at least to the wider psychiatric profession.

Weekes was a ruthless editor. Every word counted and had to be understood and assimilated easily. When a patient left the office feeling better about themselves, she claimed that '50 per cent of the job was done'. She had insisted A&R put her photo on the back cover of the book because 'so many had told her' that it mattered, that it added credibility. As a result, an older, bespectacled woman with a disciplined smile, dressed conservatively and wearing a string of pearls, stared steadily at the reader from the book's jacket.

The book opened with the dedication to her mother, followed by a single page devoted to an epigraph:

> 'Many of those who suffer from nervousness are persons
> of fine susceptibilities and delicate regard for honour,
> endowed with a feeling of duty and obligation toward
> others. Their nerves have tricked them, misled them.' —
> *Dr WR Houston*

Here was history, and Weekes' own history was hidden behind this: her debt to those insights into the mind–body connection direct from the pitiless Western Front in World War I. Dr W.R. Houston, whose quote so impressed her, was an American neurologist who spent several months working in a French hospital in WWI and witnessed firsthand the mental, as well as physical, torment. Houston's notion that it was people of 'fine sensibilities' who particularly suffered was heartening, and she imbued her book with this encouraging belief, proffered knowing the balm it offered to people with no self-esteem.

Sometimes Weekes strained to prove she believed the best, not the worst in her readers. People who had guilty thoughts were 'saintly people who struggle to banish them by fighting them, by trying not to think them'. This boosterism, along with a string of anecdotes of how others had become sick and then recovered, softened the science.

In *Self Help for Your Nerves*, Weekes identified two separate kinds of nervous illness that could 'trick people into breakdown'. First was what she called simple nervous illness, suffered by those who were hostage to fear of fear, which often followed a temporary stress or some sudden physical strain. They had become alarmed by their physical and mental symptoms. Then there were more complicated cases, where other problems perpetuated the symptoms, so Weekes had chapters on 'problems', 'sorrow', 'guilt and disgrace', and 'obsession'. She went on to cover more general difficulties such as 'sleeplessness', 'that dreaded morning feeling', and 'loss of confidence', as well as providing advice to the family.

Above all, she was practical, and made what seemed abnormal, normal. Nerves were explained medically, with useful examples. She demonstrated how the fear that felt overwhelming was limited — not even deliberate effort could make it worse, as 'the power of the adrenaline releasing nerves is limited … You cannot worsen your symptoms by facing them'.

Psychiatrists had sought for the 'why' of the suffering, over weeks, months, and years. Behaviourists flipped the coin, ignored the why, and attempted to change behaviours; one method was exposure to fears while teaching, or perhaps preaching, relaxation. Weekes' work involved exposure, too, so there was some overlap, although her protocol was quite different and did not involve training in relaxing. Passing through the panic was the way she addressed exposure.

Behaviourism morphed into cognitive behaviour therapy in

the later part of the 20th century. Dr Aaron Beck's CBT aimed at changing people's negative thought patterns, to replace them with more realistic ones, using a process called 'cognitive restructuring'.

Weekes did not give as much credit to the rational brain. Visceral fear could not be banished by appeal to higher executive functions. She had tried that herself. Anxiety impeded rational thinking. The priority therefore was to reduce the anxiety. What she also knew and saw in her surgery was that intelligent thoughtful people could be disturbed by their own thoughts. Thoughts then had power, but not in their own right. They were like the tiger that triggered the fight-or-flight reflex, only the threat was inside, an inner animal eliciting a primal response. Thoughts then, she counselled, were just that. Only thoughts. Accepting, not fighting, was again the antidote. Fighting just gave them power. Have the thoughts, she advised. Try to make them worse if you can. The objective was they not matter all.

Weekes didn't reject the idea that a change in attitude could be helpful to people, but it wasn't her primary objective, as she clearly pointed out in one of her later books. 'Although my treatment of sensitisation is based on altering the mood of the patient's approach to his condition, I am aiming at curing a definite upset in physical nervous function (heightened response) which, for convenience, I shall continue to call nervous illness.'[9]

The people who particularly, and often immediately, benefited from her work were those suffering from what had not yet been identified but would later come to be known as panic attacks. Weekes' own experience taught her that overwhelming anxiety needed urgent help, not an appointment next week with the doctor and the couch. It was the reason she always picked up the phone and never turned a sufferer away.

Although the book was a total package, Weekes saw an important role for counselling, but from some trusted source, and she warned readers to 'choose your help as carefully as you can. Let it be your wisest and not just your nearest friend.' The insoluble problem may be helped 'by an experienced counsellor ... who can teach you to look at it from a less distressing point of view'.

In the beginning, however, was 'sensitisation'. This was this process the professionals failed to understand, so could not explain to people suffering from nerves. She argued the nervous system became sensitised, either through sickness, or from the relentless worry about some problem, which primed the body to be 'tricked' by the nervous response that followed, which induced fear, which then perpetuated a vicious cycle.

The same year *Self Help for Your Nerves* was published, another psychiatrist took a step into history. Donald Klein had written a paper on a drug called imipramine after dosing 200 psychiatric patients with it, to discover serendipitously that it cut into the symptoms of panic, or what Freud called anxiety neurosis, and what Weekes called nervous illness. This drug discovery would lead to a new category of mental illness — panic disorder — but it was almost 20 years before this condition had a place in the psychiatric manual.

Weekes avoided labels, preferring the umbrella of 'nerves'. She took one therapeutic approach to any number of what would later be chopped up into different anxiety states. This set her against, and ahead of, the times. By the 1970s, the trend was to identify and label different disorders.

'A certain amount of suffering is good for us, particularly when young,' she concluded. 'We should not be sheltered too much. The experience you gain from your present suffering could be your staff in the years to come.'[10]

They were the last words in her book, yet her counsel of acceptance bore no relationship to what would be called 'tough love' years later. Acceptance worked. It was as simple as that. 'The

Chinese have a proverb expressing this. They say: "Trouble is a tunnel through which we pass and not a brick wall against which we must break our head.'"[11]

Bob DuPont identified Weekes' 'signal achievement' in *Self Help for Your Nerves* as being 'a fundamental step forward in the understanding of the treatment of anxiety disorders'. These were the most common of all mental illnesses in the world and yet 'the suffering endured by people with anxiety disorders has been made worse by the common minimisation by non-sufferers, who equate their own normal anxiety with the intense anguish of the clinically anxious person, and by the fact that many physicians, including many psychiatrists, simply do not even now understand the problems and the solutions to this disorder'.[12]

Weekes later told readers that although it seemed as if there was so much to remember, so much to do, 'there isn't you know. It is all in one word — accept.'[13] This was her central idea, which took decades to filter through to the wider profession. Forty-two years later, a textbook, *Clinical Applications of Cognitive Therapy*, gave Weekes rare acknowledgement for its provenance. 'The idea of acceptance in the treatment of Panic Disorder was introduced beautifully by Claire Weekes back in the 1960s.'[14] In the late 1980s, Weekes told her niece Frances that she believed her work would endure for another 50 years.

Chapter 19

UNSCIENTIFIC SCIENCE

Two men born in 1856 would start an argument about the mind that would rage for well over a century and remain contemporary: was there a unifying phenomenon underlying mental illness or were there a series of discrete conditions, best understood by their special differences? Sigmund Freud, born in Freiberg in Mähren, in the Austrian Empire, was what was known as a lumper, while Emil Kraepelin, from Neustrelitz, Germany, was a splitter. The year after both were born, Charles Darwin wrote to his friend the botanist J.D. Hooker making a distinction between the two different scholarly approaches, concluding that both were needed. 'It is good to have hair-splitters and lumpers,' he wrote in 1857.[1]

Known as the 'great German psychiatric classifier', Kraepelin judged that psychoanalysis was 'not sufficiently based on scientific principles' and sought to name and identify specific psychiatric conditions.[2] His legacy lived on, and the same battle would be enjoined in the 1970s in another even more bloody engagement with the Freudians. Kraepelin and his heirs stood for measurement and empiricism whereas Freud's psychoanalytic approach seemed to owe as much to art as science.

That was one big arena, but there were plenty of other

significant campaigns. When Weekes wrote *Self Help for Your Nerves* with her focus on the nervous system in the early 1960s, among the competitors to the Freudians were the Radical Behaviourists, led by Harvard psychiatrist B.F. Skinner. Behaviourism dated back to the earlier theories of the American psychologist John Watson, who, in 1912, was prosecuting the case for relying on observable behaviour only, and sidelining thoughts and feelings. Where Freudians dived into the depths of the unconscious, behaviourists ignored the unobservable in favour of what could be seen, the behaviour.

This was another iteration of the battle for a science of the mind, and Watson's theory was another intellectual rebuke of psychoanalytic introspection — it wouldn't be the last. Still, there were plenty of critics of behaviourism and its 'mechanistic approach', and his contemporary, the psychologist William McDougall, chided him for relying on 'data of one kind only, the data or facts of observation obtainable by observing the movements and other bodily changes exhibited by human and other organisms'.[3]

Watson's work followed that of Ivan Pavlov, a Russian physiologist who trained dogs to salivate at the ringing of a bell. From Pavlov came the notion that behaviour was learned, or conditioned. What could be learned could be unlearned. Pavlov coined the concept of 'nervism' and linked it particularly to the gastrointestinal tract.

Building on the theories and experiments of Pavlov and Watson, Skinner's concepts of positive and negative reinforcement supported his proposition that the environment shaped the human. Again, it was based on observable behaviour alone, though the results of Skinner's experiments on rats were extrapolated to people.[4]

While psychoanalysis proved incapable of being supported by empiricism, the behaviourists endeavoured to establish a scientific and statistical support for their work on the troubled mind. Weekes stood outside these battles, her methodology having been fostered by a biological approach, with its historic preoccupation with the connection between the mind and the body. In the middle of the 20th century, attempts were made to integrate biology with psychology and the physiological regulation of emotion. The complex pathways — psychological, neurological, and hormonal — were being explored as a 'science' in laboratories, and in clinical settings.[5] Freudian psychoanalysis continued to find favour, but doctors and scientists tended towards a biological view of mental suffering.

There was no better example of this than the Hungarian-Canadian doctor Hans Selye, a leading authority on endocrinology, among other medical specialties, who wrote his first 'stress' monograph in 1950 and was credited with anointing the word that became a metaphor for modern life. Selye's landmark work, *The Stress of Life*, showed, as Weekes would later demonstrate herself in her work, the way in which stress induced hormonal autonomic responses. Selye then identified how these could lead to serious diseases, such as ulcers, high blood pressure, arteriosclerosis, arthritis, and kidney disease.

Into this mix of approaches — Freudian, behavioural, biological — came the allure of drugs. As Weekes treated her patients with explanations of how the nervous system worked, and how it could be managed, pharmaceutical companies were funding research for a pill that would take mental pain away, encouraged by the recent discovery of a new class of drugs that calmed agitation. Yet so little was known of brain chemistry in the 1950s that those drugs had been discovered quite by accident, a serendipitous by-product of medications designed to treat other conditions.[6]

Gavin Andrews, Australia's pre-eminent specialist in anxiety and a professor of psychiatry at the University of New South

Wales in Sydney, says that when he graduated as a doctor, in 1956, he believed the biochemistry of mental disorders was about to be unravelled. 'For the first time, we had drugs for anxiety, depression, and madness, and expected this would be the start of them in psychiatry, and believed that within ten years there would be parallels with the treatment of diabetes — we would find an insulin for the mind.'

Money was poured into pharmacological research into antidepressants, which were developed for humans based on experiments on rats.

It's not hard to see why Weekes infuriated the professionals, according to Andrews. 'Here was a lady saying don't take barbiturates, which were the sedatives of the day, and I'm sure doctors found her challenging because she did not think much of the way they treated people. She challenged the orthodoxy of the medical profession, which was embracing for the first time the antidepressant drugs, anti-anxiety drugs, and antipsychotics as drugs. Here was this lady saying, there's a better way to do it.'

By the early 1960s, the mental-health profession was atomised between psychiatrists and psychologists, between those who believed in drugs and those who didn't. Did you treat the whole person or a set of genes? Did you plumb the unconscious or did you try to change behaviour? How do you change people's attitudes and therefore their moods?

Weekes wasn't winning friends in any circles. She regarded Freudian psychoanalysis as a waste of time, and, although attitude and patterns of thinking were important, they ran second to her emphasis on the nervous system. As for the behaviourist's desensitisation, she thought an understanding of *sensitisation* was a better route to understanding anxiety, and she never preached relaxation, as it could be so unrelaxing in practice. Finally, while there was some virtue in occasional, modest sedation, her objective was to have people living independently of medication.

The same year that Weekes published her book, the psychologist Albert Ellis — considered along with Aaron Beck to be one of the main originators of the so-called cognitive revolution in psychology[7] — wrote *Reason and Emotion in Psychotherapy*, ushering in cognitive therapy, which would be blended into behaviour therapy. Now thoughts mattered, along with behaviour. Where Ellis saw irrationality, Beck saw inaccurate thinking — but both worked at changing the way people thought about themselves, and the world around them. CBT, of which Ellis' Rational Emotive Behaviour Therapy was the first form, would come to define modern psychology.

Yet Ellis had a high opinion of the work of Weekes. Professor Raymond DiGiuseppe, who worked with Ellis from 1975 until Ellis' death, says, 'Al Ellis used to talk about her work when I was a postdoctoral fellow in the 1970s. We would regularly refer/ recommend the books by Dr Weekes for clients. Bibliotherapy was a big part of REBT and Dr Weekes's books were at the top of the recommended reading list as long as the books were available.'

Weekes would later be identified as a precursor to CBT, yet her approach involved a package of ideas that did not fit neatly into that box. Changing how you thought about things, replacing negative thoughts with positive thoughts, was not her approach, although she certainly acknowledged that attitude was important, and that thoughts could have an impact on the nervous system. Yet she reversed the order of importance. Treat the nervous system first and the thoughts second. Ellis, a large charismatic New Yorker with a willingness to have his own dogmas challenged, would come to understand this himself in later years and would publicly acknowledge the work of Weekes, particularly the idea of the fear of fear.[8]

Accepting that a sensitised nervous system could not be

controlled, Weekes' advice was to 'float past' disturbing thoughts and give them no power. They were just thoughts. Her advocacy of non-reactivity, or masterly inactivity, was then quite a foreign notion. Hers was a unique therapeutic approach.

The decade after she died, another iteration of CBT was popularised by Professor Steven Hayes from the University of Nevada. It was called acceptance and commitment therapy, and had more in common with her approach, given its emphasis on acceptance. ACT has been called the third wave of CBT, and offers another example of her pioneering approach.

The '60s and early '70s ushered in the anti-psychiatry movement — a movement within psychiatry itself — and there was a growing loss of confidence in Freudian psychoanalysis. Psychoanalysts, the lumpers, found themselves under direct assault from the splitters, the neo-Kraepelins who cast themselves as more 'scientific' and championed the careful observation of symptoms in order to more fully classify and identify mental illness. The splitters became labellers who divided up several loose components in the basket of mental illness into individual disorders.

There was a century of building, tearing down, and rebuilding, and, by the 1980s, CBT had seized the day, although its own statistical claims to success were themselves contested. Strict statistical measurement of the efficacy of therapies treating the muddy waters of despair required a superhuman divining rod.

Over the years, it became clearer that drugs were not an unmitigated success, that psychoanalysis could cause as much harm as good, and that so-called behaviour therapy, or exposure of the kind championed by Dr Joseph Wolpe, had limitations in relation to one group that was proving refractory to this approach. Members of that group suffered panic attacks, especially when experiencing the great outdoors or public spaces.

Agoraphobia had no clinical profile at all until 1980, when

the labellers gained the upper hand in the psych wars and it was listed in the third edition of the *Diagnostic and Statistical Manual of Mental Disorders* (*DSM*). This was the professional psychiatric manual that defined mental disorders, and it came to underpin the legal and regulatory framework around mental illness. It offered benchmarks upon which to base an industry response. The *DSM* — which classified and measured — offered an implicit claim to scientific validity.

Weekes wrote about a landscape that she understood well. She had traversed it in her own life, and in her surgery she had extended her understanding. Although there were plenty of varieties of suffering, Weekes remained a lumper, not a splitter. They were variations on one theme: fear.

She inherited no psychiatric or psychological tradition, she followed no ideology or school of thought. If her analysis was not entirely new and was supported by the medical science of the nervous system, then no one had told the story to the public in quite the same way. And the professionals had no treatment protocol that they could prove worked. This lack of empirical results would continue to tear psychiatry apart.

Chapter 20

GETTING A GRIP ON
THE MARKET

On 26 December 1962, *Self Help for Your Nerves* was boosted by publicity money couldn't buy. *The Australian Women's Weekly* gave it a prime plug — the book's title was prominent on the magazine's front cover, and the story itself was the opening two-page spread.[1]

It opened with Weekes' memory of a male patient 'in such a state of tension through nerves that he was unable to walk or feed himself'. It was a story of a miracle recovery. He had learned to 'float' past the fear, she said, and was soon feeding himself and walking unaided up and down the hospital ward.

She used the idea of an inner voice that could be cultivated, particularly when panic returned. Each section of the feature was headlined by her simple treatment protocol: 'Facing ...' 'Accepting ...' 'Floating ...' 'And Letting Time Pass'.

There was a breakout box called '14 Do's and Dont's'. This was a crisp cheat sheet of her work.

1. Don't run away from fear.
2. Accept all the strange sensations connected with

your breakdown, recognise them as temporary.

3. Let there be no self-pity.

4. Settle your problem as quickly as you can, if not with action, then by accepting a new point of view.

5. Waste no time on 'what might have been' and 'if only'.

6. Face sorrow and know that time will bring relief.

7. Be occupied. Don't lie in bed brooding. Be occupied calmly, not feverishly trying to forget yourself.

8. Remember that the strength in the muscle may depend on the confidence with which it is used.

9. Accept your obsessions and be prepared to live with them temporarily. Do not fight them by trying to push them away. Let time do that.

10. Remember your recovery doesn't necessarily depend 'entirely on you' as so many people are ready to help you. You may need help. Accept it willingly, without shame.

11. Don't be discouraged if you cannot make decisions while you are ill. When you're well it will be easy enough to make decisions.

12. Don't measure your progress day by day. Don't count the months, years you have been ill and be dispirited at the thought of them. Once you're on the road to recovery, recovery is inevitable however protracted your illness may have been.

13. Never accept defeat. Remember it is never too late to give yourself another chance.

14. Face, accept, float, and let time pass. If you do this, you must get well.

No one could paraphrase Dr Claire Weekes better than Dr Claire Weekes. Even her publisher recognised she was her own best editor, and so the *Women's Weekly* reporter, Winifred Munday, had little to do but introduce the author and then add 'said the author' or 'Dr Weekes warns', filling up the two pages with direct quotes.

While her books were not political, Weekes' own views of gender roles, and the damage done by them, was easy to discern in her descriptions of the lot of the 1960s wife. She had no reverence for housework and gave blunt advice about this. Find something else to do, she would counsel. 'Housework is rarely interesting to a woman with a breakdown, and since interest is the force that will lift you back to normal, find it if we reasonably can.'

Instead of housework, Weekes suggested finding creative occupation, but something not demanding too much concentration. She regularly met resistance. 'It is sometimes difficult to convince a husband that it is better for his wife to attend a class in making artificial flowers than to be home cooking his dinner … His attitude is often: "if she can fill in time with flowers, why can't she cook supper?"'

Weekes understood why. She had never wanted to cook herself. 'If you are a nervously sick housewife, do not feel guilty if you want to leave the dishes, make artificial flowers, breed dogs, or dig in the garden,' she said.

There were more reviews, and good ones from some serious publications such as the *Australian Book Review*. 'Most of us have been brought to a point of total cynicism about books which constitute help yourself psychiatry, but once one starts to read this book all ugly suspicions disappear. It has a particular excellence which is certainly not to be found in all available USA books in the field.'

Brisk sales of *Self Help for Your Nerves* meant Weekes, at the age of 59, was sufficiently confident in her future to retire from full-time medical practice in 1963, although she would remain a consultant physician at Rachel Forster Hospital. Nevertheless, while the book was immediately and gratifyingly successful, it became obvious early on that, in this field, popularity and professional respect were mutually exclusive.

The psychiatric community was either uninterested or critical, but her peers in the medical profession were more receptive — she was one of theirs, after all. Not long after publication, *The Medical Journal of Australia* reviewed *Self Help for Your Nerves* and advised 'it can be recommended as a prescription with the physician's blessing ... Much of it could be annotated "read t.d.s. [*ter die sumendum*: three times daily] with advantage to the patient".'[2] Her advice was a better alternative to medication, the journal concluded. Weekes could not have wished for more comprehensive validation from a journal with reach throughout the community.

The year after *Self Help for Your Nerves* was published, Roche Lab launched Valium on the market as one in a new drug class called benzodiazepines, which included Librium, Klonopin, and Xanax. These were sedatives, with addictive power. Then came the antidepressants. The idea of chemical imbalance in the brain was starting to take hold. Never mind that drug efficacy was often a serendipitous accident. The chemical-imbalance theory would become increasingly powerful over the years, as psychoanalysis and psychological treatments struggled. Drugs offered a potential magic bullet.

Given the hit or miss of medication, some doctors came to see Weekes' books as a better alternative. However, she remained up against Freud, and an impenetrable citadel of professional belief. 'When I first began to work, Freudian analysis was still the treatment of choice for the anxiety state, including agoraphobia, and so many people are not only not helped by this, some were actually harmed, and some of these came to me to be rescued.'

The news of her success continued to spread among the medical profession. As they saw their patients were helped by her books, doctors would recommend them to others, and so the books were promoted informally.

The reception for *Self Help for Your Nerves* in Australia suggested real potential for export, and the book was published by Angus & Robertson in the UK and then (as *Hope and Help for Your Nerves*) by Coward-McCann in the US in 1963. In the same year, a Viennese-born psychiatrist and scholar, Dr Trudy Spencer, came across Weekes' work. Spencer had trained as a psychiatrist in Washington and spent five years there. She wrote Weekes an admiring letter on official letterhead and warned of how difficult it could be to get 'recognition in America'.

'I know perfectly well what you are up against. I did my psychiatry in Washington, DC and spent five years there in a very Freudian environment. Those circles will be very difficult to penetrate, as everything new and contrary to the old is rejected. It's the old story.'

Writing to Weekes, Spencer had enclosed a copy of a paper she had written on Shoma Morita, a Japanese psychiatrist whom she described as 'practically a contemporary of Freud'. Morita had devised an extensive method to treat a type of anxiety neurosis the Japanese called *shinkeishitu*, wrote Spencer. 'There is a great similarity between your technique and his, and I find this coincidence remarkable.'

Central to Morita's theory 'is the observation of thoughts, feelings and body sensations that are uncontrollable through an act of will. The successful student of Morita therapy is to be aware of and accept the moment to moment fluctuations of thoughts and feelings without unnecessary struggle or resistance.'[3] Or put another way, Morita 'sees the healing of the patients not in the removal of their fears but in the inner acceptance of the fears they have experienced'.[4]

Spencer said she would be most interested in Weekes' opinion of the theory. What Weekes thought of it is unknown; however, she kept Spencer's letter for 25 years. In one respect, Spencer predicted the future, concluding her letter with some hope: 'America is an enlightened country in many ways and has given birth to many new and revolutionary things, and it is not impossible at all that you will be able to make yourself heard.'

By the mid-1960s *Self Help for Your Nerves* was selling well enough for A&R to plan paperback editions in Australia and Britain. In 1966, Weekes signed a new contract. Her editor, Beatrice Davis, was respectful of her doctor-author status, ensuring that Weekes was intimately involved in the publicity for the paperbacks and approved any endorsements on the cover. Among those selected by Weekes was one from the *Daily Sketch*, London: 'A remarkable adventure in human understanding that can help you live on top of the world.'

On the surface, all was well, but, behind the scenes, Weekes was struggling with her agent, Inky Stephensen. He finally had the promise of a bestseller, but their relationship had broken down. Like anything to do with Stephensen's finances, and typical of Weekes' subsequent dealings with male advocates for her work, it ended messily. Even more typically, the mess continued to fester, never being properly resolved. If A&R had been paying attention, the first sign that not all was well between the pair was when Stephensen wrote instructing the publisher to pay 90 per cent of all monies earned direct to her and just credit him with his 10 per cent agent's commission. Weekes had wrestled back control of her payments. That was the first step.

On 21 October 1964, she officially terminated his 'agency agreement'. Stephensen no longer represented her, but Weekes said nothing to A&R, who, unaware of her decision, continued to pay Stephensen his 10 per cent commission. Weekes never cancelled it. She did not like conflict, and Stephensen was nothing if not volatile.

Yet Stephensen would get barely two years' worth of royalty payments from *Self Help for Your Nerves*. On 29 June 1965, he was guest speaker at the annual Australian Literature Night, which was held by the Savage Club in the State Ballroom in Market Street, Sydney. 'Stephensen spoke brilliantly about book censorship and his part in the secret London edition of *Lady Chatterley's Lover*,' according to Craig Munro. 'The members of the Savage Club gave him a standing ovation ... After the applause from the members of the Savage Club had died away, Stephensen rose again, thanked them, and fell dead in his seat.'[5]

After his death, Weekes took the opportunity to claim back the royalty payments Stephensen had received after she ended their relationship in 1964. She put her lawyers, A.E. McIntosh & Henderson and B.J. Moroney, on the case, and they wrote to 'The Manager, Angus & Robertson' on 29 October 1965, a few months later.

As a doctor, Weekes controlled her own affairs. Now there were literary agents, publishers, and, eventually, motley entrepreneurs to wrangle. They would prove far more disappointing than grateful patients. First there had been the excitable Stephensen, now there was a bureaucracy. Her lawyers hit an institutional wall, and there was no response to their letter, and so, in January 1966, they wrote again. Weekes' statement for the period 1 January 1965 to 30 June 1965 showed deductions for 'both domestic and overseas royalties' that she presumed 'were credited to the account of Mr P R Stephensen'.[6] Her lawyers respectfully demanded 'that any amounts which have been deducted for agency fees due to the late Mr Stephensen be paid to Dr Weekes forthwith'.

When A&R finally responded, Weekes' lawyers were astonished to find, instead of a resolution, they had been sent a copy of *Self Help for Your Nerves* with an invoice for $2.87 (the pound having being replaced by the dollar on 14 February 1966). They sent it back to the publisher. 'The book is returned herewith and we would appreciate your reply to our letter of October 29, 1965.'

A frustrated Weekes wrote to her efficient editor, hoping

Davis could sort it out. Stephensen had 'ceased being my agent in 1964', she wrote, adding that it was 'because of certain personal reasons' and the 'matter is more complicated than this but we need not go into it'. Despite this, Weekes had 'allowed him to continue receiving his royalty until the time of his death', but added that 'death cancels all contracts'.

Davis had her own history with Stephensen and organised an apologetic letter to Weekes' lawyers on 25 May 1966, explaining that somehow the Accounts Department had not known of the final instruction from Weekes cancelling his payment after his death. Davis advised them that A&R would pay Weekes a cheque for £23.58 for the last royalty period, covering the amount that had been credited to Stephensen's account, and reassured them that all future royalties would be paid in full to Weekes.

To Weekes herself, she wrote with a hint of irritation about Stephensen.

> Dear Dr Weekes,
>
> Just to acknowledge your helpful letter of 17 May, and to say that we shall be putting the paperback edition in hand straight away, and also preparing the leaflet. What a pity you didn't officially tell us that P.R. Stephensen ceased to be your agent in 1964, although you allowed him to receive his share of royalties until the time of his death. I don't know whether the 10% deducted from your July–December cheque was sent to Stephensen's widow, but I shall investigate this with Mr Iliffe and let you know how things stand.[7]

Davis subsequently sent a memo to 'Iliffe' where she pointed out the overpayment to 'P.R. Stephensen' and concluded: 'Please remember that all future earnings on *Self Help*, whether from Sydney or London sales, or on foreign additional royalties are to be paid in full to Dr Weekes.' She underlined the two words 'in full'. The memos shot around A&R. No royalties were to be paid to the Estate of P.R. Stephensen, 'which will apply to foreign monies that may come through London'.[8] After the matter was resolved, one of Weekes' lawyers, who had returned her book to A&R, noted dryly that their 'salesmanship is to be admired if not their efficiency'.

By 1965, Weekes was spending a significant amount of time in London and proving her own best publicist. She was enjoying being back in Europe and travelling again. The book was out in the US, and she was particularly happy with the reviews reprinted on the jacket of that edition and was looking forward to the paperback edition. Excited by the book's success, she fretted about A&R's marketing competence. She anticipated a tidal wave of demand in the UK, and restlessly worried the London office had no inkling of this and were therefore unprepared.

In May 1966, she wrote several letters to Davis about the proposed paperback. She particularly wanted Davis to understand the 'coming sales boost to the book in England', and urged her politely to produce 'a new edition as soon as possible'. She pointed out that there was a forthcoming article in *She* magazine, as well as ones in *Woman*, *The Nurses Quarterly*, and the *Journal of the Mental Health Organisation, England*. There was more.

> As well as this, the Open Door Association in England and Scotland is making purchase of the book one of the conditions of membership and this association is growing rapidly. It has increased from 250 members to 2250 in one year and with the coming publicity should increase still further.

This was a breakthrough. The Open Door was established in 1959 by a long-suffering agoraphobic, Alice Neville from Chislehurst, Kent, who had cured herself by doing the very things she feared the most. Neville had been most impressed with *Self Help for Your Nerves*, and she and Weekes had forged a mutually beneficial relationship.

Despite Weekes' misgivings about A&R, her relationship with Davis remained good. She met all of Weekes' requests. 'It is splendid to know there is such great prospects for *Self Help* in the UK, and we know that the London office will do their utmost to take advantage of the publicity.'

By now, other countries were interested in the book, and Weekes was typically hands-on. In one of the European editions, she had insisted on changing the translation of her word 'float'. The translator had other ideas and was determined to win the argument, but for all the right reasons: he loved the book. On 3 July 1965, he wrote to Weekes in Australia to argue his case and reveal that behind his professional judgement lay a personal story. This was typical — even when Weekes wasn't targeting an audience, she would find one.

The translator introduced himself and said he had 'two reasons' to write to her. To begin with, he wanted to thank her for writing her book, but then disclosed that he was possibly the first person in his country to make use of her advice. 'I have never had a nervous breakdown, but I certainly had "bad nerves" at the end of last year, when I received your book,' he wrote. The translator then explained that his heart had been troubling him for a couple of years, but her explanation had cleared up the problem almost completely. However, the greater part of his gratitude was for the way in which the book helped his wife.

My wife was actually in hospital with a bad nervous breakdown when I received your book. She has been ill for about 15 years and spent many months in various hospitals. She has had shock treatment, continuous sedation et cetera and was slightly improved but never really cured. I need not explain to you what her life was like; she was sometimes on the verge of throwing it away. I had given up all hope myself, and I think that her illness was perhaps partly to blame for my own troubles. The worst of it was that I could not understand her and felt so utterly helpless.

When she was released from the hospital, I gave her the manuscript of the translation to read. Now for the first time, she feels she can get out of the troubles. She still has many setbacks, but she knows the way and I know now I can help her. She is already much better. She has even taken up a part-time job and this is something that would have seemed impossible a year ago. I also hope the publishers will be able to give the book the publicity it deserves. (It is a pity you did not give it to a more prominent publishing firm.)

He argued that the word he preferred had a 'positive and more specific character and was a single intransitive verb like "float"', and hoped she would permit him his choice, as, he said, 'the very sound of it has a comforting relaxing effect'.[9]

By the end of 1966, Weekes was fretting about the competence of the London office, and the efforts of the London manager, Walter Butcher. Davis was confident Butcher knew how well the book was received in England and would ensure there were adequate stocks to meet the demand. Weekes could not be convinced and wrote to Butcher herself. 'Dear Mr Butcher, you will have probably noticed that my book is beginning to sell well in England at last'.

Weekes pointed to the endorsement of her book by the Open Door, which she described as the mental-health equivalent of Alcoholics Anonymous. She did not want Butcher to be in any doubt about her growing popularity, telling him that the organiser, Neville, had received 'hundreds of letters' praising the monthly articles Weekes had written for their journal. 'Indeed, the suffering people say they have never read or heard anything like them. So, you see my name will gradually come to be known throughout the UK. I will certainly see that it is.'

She urged Butcher to contact Neville to assess demand, as the association had 'a huge waiting list and only six copies in the library. From my experience, once a person borrows this book and returns it, he or she almost always orders a copy for themselves.' Neville wanted to promote her book, she told him. 'I have told her she is at liberty to say whatever she wishes. It is only I who must not talk in that way.'

Weekes threw in at the end of the letter that 'Miss Davis is alert and with your cooperation, I am sure will see that enough books are ready to meet any increased demand.' This suggested that Davis herself may have encouraged Weekes to write directly to Butcher.

Weekes was right to anticipate that London would struggle to meet demand. On 1 January 1967, Davis sent a memo to George Ferguson letting him know of the 'tremendous publicity for herself [Weekes] and the book — particularly a long article in the Sunday Mirror'. However, 'apparently London has been unable to supply for some months because, though the bound books arrived, the jackets were for paperback'. Weekes was beside herself.

Back in the Sydney office, Davis asked Ferguson 'when will the right jackets reach London? Dr Weekes said she begged WB

[Walter Butcher] to sell the books without jackets when the big demand was on. Did he do this?'

Later that year, Ferguson sent out a group memo under the heading 'Weekes: Self Help For Your Nerves'. 'Please note that London Office have a suddenly increased demand for this book and are going to reprint a litho [lithographically reproduced] edition for their own market.'

Now they discovered for themselves what Weekes knew — *Self Help for Your Nerves* was taking off. Davis asked Ferguson to make sure that the book got a push in South Africa. By May 1966, it had been translated and sold into France, Germany, the Netherlands, Denmark, and Norway.[10] There were requests from publishers in South Africa, Japan, India, Israel, and Italy.

Soon royalty cheques were arriving from all over the world. Some of them would go astray, and so Weekes learned to keep a closer eye on her originating publisher. She discovered that the literary agent Robert Harben, who was handling foreign sales for A&R, had sent a royalty cheque worth £144 to the Sydney office for sales of the Dutch edition, but the cheque had not made it to her bank account. She wrote to the A&R accountant about this, requesting payment, and noted Walter Butcher had another royalty cheque for sales in England for the first six months of 1968 that was due to her. 'Would you kindly see it is also sent to my address at Macquarie Street as soon as possible? It is for a considerable amount, nearly $4000, so you would appreciate that I would like delivery soon.'

The response in England and Europe augured well for an even bigger market: the US. 'She is now off to America to do further talking and advertising of S.Help,' her editor said in a memo to Ferguson.

Yet while Weekes toured the US, things were unravelling back in Cremorne. Dulcie rattled around the downstairs apartment, her labile moods inadequately managed by medication. She was now under pressure from her brother Brian to care for the two children from his second marriage, ten-year-old Barbara and 14-year-old Tim. He wanted his wife Esther to be free to accompany him on his travels, finding them unbearably lonely by himself. Dulcie agreed to look after her niece and nephew for three months.

Tim and Barbara didn't know what had hit them. The arrangement was a disaster, and there was no Weekes to help sort it out. Dulcie spent most of the time in bed, and the children found themselves either in the middle of a wider family drama or left alone. Barbara wrote to her mother: 'God I hate it here, there's never anybody around ...' The letters convinced Brian and Esther that Dulcie wasn't coping. Tim and Barbara were dispatched to other relatives, although it meant far longer travelling times to school.

Weekes, the 'fixer-upperer' as her niece Tita called her, was never very effective at 'fixing' her own family. Lili pointed to the occupational paradox: the painter's house was never painted; the plumber's taps dripped. Or as Tita put it: no woman is a prophet in her own home.

Chapter 21

A SECOND HOME

Weekes' work, now focused on her books, had also become a bridge to new friendships, many of which were built on gratitude. This was her path to the elegant, emotionally fragile London magistrate Joyce Skene Keating, which would become, beyond her relationship with Coleman, one of the closest bonds in Weekes' life. The two women met at the Open Door, which Skene Keating had joined seeking help for her agoraphobia.

Skene Keating rapidly fell under the spell of the Australian doctor with her promise of a cure, her utter confidence in the possibility of recovery, and her practical approach to nervous illness. As Weekes was spending extended periods in London spruiking her work, she had taken Skene Keating on as a patient, who therein discovered the unqualified commitment that 'treatment' from this Australian doctor entailed.

Skene Keating had her own unqualified offering in return. Weekes, or 'Weekey' as she would be called by the Skene Keating family, found a permanent home in Kensington in their central city apartment. With its two floors, seven bedrooms, several reception areas, lofty ceilings, and view over a large garden square, it was spacious and comfortable.

Skene Keating's husband had died several years earlier, and she had two young children, Paul and Julia, as well as a live-in nanny, Irene Appleton, affectionately known as 'Nan'. The flat in the five-storey Victorian dwelling at 33 Queen's Gate Gardens became a second home for Weekes over the following decades, and she made extensive use of it, usually with Coleman in tow.

This was the first of several such intimate arrangements, although few had the personal intensity of the one Weekes shared with Skene Keating. Weekes made no effort to keep a professional distance from her patients, and everywhere in the world there would be someone to stay with who, one way or another, was beholden to her work, and happy to offer their hospitality or their services. There was never any shortage of thoughtful, intelligent, suffering individuals who regarded her as a genius, as well as a friend, which well suited a woman who loved companionship.

In the mid-1960s, a memo lobbed onto the desk of Beatrice Davis: 'Dr Weekes wanted to be sure (the other day) that you have this address to reach her in London. C/o Mrs Skene Keating, JP. 33 Queensgate Gardens. London SW7.'

From 1964 onwards, Weekes increasingly spent much of the year here, as well as in the US. She relished international travel. London was a good base, and Skene Keating put no limits on her hospitality. She was Weekes' host, patient, and friend. This tall, finely boned woman who had long struggled with agoraphobia found some real and early relief from the treatment she received from Weekes, but the 'cure' did not necessarily grow with proximity nor last the distance of their relationship. Skene Keating remained a highly stressed individual, although her agoraphobia did improve, according to her son.

As Weekes spent so much time living with the Skene Keatings, they became known to Weekes' wider family, who would visit from time to time. When Weekes was in London, her accent became what her niece Penny called AEAP, or *As English As Possible*. Once Penny visited Weekes at the Kensington apartment, accompanied by her Skarratt grandmother, whose English poise had always slightly discomfited her other grandmother, Fan.

The blinds were pulled and the house was dark and the hired help bought in the afternoon tea. At the end of the visit, Penny and her grandmother left the apartment accompanied by Weekes. They walked down a long set of stairs into the sunshine outside, where the farewells became extended. Weekes walked up the street with her relatives. Eventually, they heard Skene Keating anxiously calling out for Weekes, uncertain of her whereabouts. Weekes returned to Skene Keating, and, a little further down the street Penny's grandmother looked over her shoulder and in her clipped English, using her pet name for her granddaughter, said: 'Well, Popsy, that doesn't look like a cure to me!'

In London, Weekes replicated the hierarchy she enjoyed in Sydney. Skene Keating was dependent and passionately devoted. Nan's support of Weekes would later be rewarded with a dedication in one of her books. All Weekes' physical needs were attended to, and Coleman blended into the background, providing a support role. The situation was less satisfactory for the two children of the household, who felt invisible when their mother's great friend was staying. At dinnertime, Weekes and Skene Keating were consumed with themselves and the children were ignored. Weekes was not a natural with children in any case, and Paul and Julia were not family, they just came with Skene Keating.

Still, given the time Weekes and Coleman spent with them, the two children got to know the two women well. Paul Skene Keating's respect and admiration for the work of Weekes is unambiguous. As an adult, he trained as a musician, and later as a therapist himself. He regards her as a pioneer, her work as unique, and he saw firsthand her enormous public profile in Britain.

'Everybody, regardless of any sort of status, social and financial, knew who she was. Everybody knew about her in this country!'

What Paul also remembers are the 'literally sackfuls of mail'. Her books advertised her other resources, such as her audio cassettes and records, and gave the Skene Keating home as the contact address. The local post office struggled to cope with the landslide of letters, and Paul and Julia occasionally had to collect the 'sacks' themselves.

Then there were the people who would ring, and sometimes just turn up. A pilot who had developed a phobia serious enough to ground him arrived at the house without warning. He had spent a fortune seeking help because his passion, as well as his income, was in aviation. 'In a very short period, I think we're talking six months, Claire had sorted him. And I was really impressed as he had been ill for a very long time and yet he got his job back again,' says Paul.

He wasn't the only one she got back into the air. On 24 April 1971, a telegram addressed to Weekes arrived at 33 Queen's Gate Gardens.

> I read your book. I listened to your records. I made a call to you. I'm a new person. I fly in small aircraft and it's great to be alive again.
> (name withheld) Tehachapi California.

There was a pop star with stage fright whom Weekes returned to the limelight. Weekes herself in a speech in later years referred to 'the famous people, you'd know some of them if I told you the names' who had come to her for help.[1]

As he witnessed the power of her work, Paul was astonished that a woman of such intelligence chose his mother and a bunch of other patients around the world to handle the audio and video side of her business, and in such a ragtag fashion. 'Here was a woman, who is a genius, who is writing these extraordinary books way ahead of their time, and is relying on vulnerable patients rather than employing professionals,' he observes. Paul notes that there always seemed to be trouble with some patient she had hooked up with commercially.

It was a pattern she never broke. Dr Zane at the White Plains phobia clinic had successfully turned his recovered patients into therapists at the hospital, yet that was quite a different proposition from inviting them to run a distribution business. Given the demand for her audiotapes, and all the mail that arrived from England, Skene Keating had a real administrative burden, which she bore graciously out of devotion to Weekes. Paul remembers just how much work was put in by his mother, but also by Nan and Coleman. 'It was hard graft, and they were dedicated, efficient, and loyal,' he says.

Paul thinks *Self Help for Your Nerves* was seminal, 'a staggering book'. Yet the puzzle was not just Weekes' misguided business instincts but the woman herself. He judges that her ability to relate to others was circumscribed. Her interpersonal success did not extend as well to those who fell outside her arena of professional interests. He accepts that perhaps this came with the territory, and reaches the same conclusion as some other members of her family. To be as good as she was required drive and self-possession, if not obsession. Weekes could be autocratic and self-centred, and Paul, like others, witnessed her imperiousness.

There were, however, glimpses of the lighter Weekes side — for instance, when she shared holidays with the Skene Keatings: photos show an older woman laughing on a swing, sitting on a toboggan, but such frivolous pleasures were rare.

While Weekes remained the sun around which the planets moved, there was one big difference from home life in Australia.

In London, Coleman was finally visible. Within the Skene Keating family, she was not only seen but heard and deeply appreciated — by Paul and Julia. As they struggled for their own place in the home when Weekes was around, Paul noticed how difficult it was for Coleman, too. 'The relationship between my mum and Claire was very strong. I think Beth was very much sidelined,' he says. Paul felt this keenly, and became very attached to Coleman, who paid sensitive attention to him and to his younger sister. Of the two Australian women, it was Coleman for whom Paul reserved his unqualified affection. He gave his own daughter 'Beth' as a middle name, a tribute to a woman he describes as 'deeply moral'. Always interested in music, he also recognises that Coleman, while completely overshadowed by Weekes, had an extraordinary talent in her own right.

'She was an absolutely ace concert pianist, I mean we are talking phenomenal, phenomenal.' Yet beyond her brilliance as a pianist was something else Paul valued even more. What became obvious to him was a quality of character in Coleman that remained unseen back in Australia. The young boy, and the young man he became, who was missing a father and had a self-obsessed mother, found in Coleman the empathy he craved. She offered a real quality of attention. Coleman had, Paul says with intensity, 'really, really good listening skills. She would have made an absolutely *brilliant* counsellor.'

Coleman, he says, would just dive in. She would listen, reflect, and respond with something genuinely pertinent and helpful, full of common sense. This was a side of Coleman unseen by the Weekes family, but it was always available to Weekes herself.

'Of the two of them, Beth was very warm and very soft and very well-intentioned, and Claire was full-on with her work, so almost anything extramural got in the way,' he says. However, Paul appreciates that as a professional woman, Weekes would have struggled to get recognition in that era.

The pressures on Weekes, and her self-absorption, meant she hit the wrong note in her personal life from time to time. The woman who spoke with such authority and compassion to distraught strangers for hours on the phone could be insensitive when not fully engaged. One day, a youth she knew well came to her in distress, about to get married but concerned it was to the wrong person. Either because she could not be bothered, or because she decided it might stray into some uncomfortable sexual terrain, Weekes spectacularly missed the point and snapped the door closed with an inappropriate aphorism: 'All black cats are the same in the night.' It was a piece of biological reductionism that was never forgotten, and she was never asked for advice from that quarter again.

Chapter 22

BAD BUSINESS

At the age of 65, Weekes saw her first book return to the bestseller list in Britain after five years on the market, achieving that ranking more than once in 1968. 'I believe this made publication history,' Weekes said.[1] Her work was reaching a mass market.

On 16 February 1969, she was a guest on prime-time BBC, following the six o'clock news, on a program called *Living with One's Fears*.[2] Along with the press coverage, her audience was growing. By April 1969, Weekes was contracted with Hawthorn Books in the US for a paperback edition, and she embarked on coast-to-coast promotional tours.

Weekes was elated. She was in demand in Britain and America and relishing it, being treated, at least in the popular press, as the expert she knew herself to be. 'No patient has ever told me of a fear of which I hadn't heard before,' she regularly observed.[3]

Her indomitable mood was captured in one report that had her 'laughing, her blue-green eyes sparkling' as she declared that 'at my age, 66, you don't have any real fears. I have even become reconciled to my future.'[4]

Weekes' work anticipated a modern approach to mental health. She dismissed negative stereotypes of nervous illness before this became more acceptable. So many nervously afflicted people were 'ordinary people with no particular personality problem'. Psychiatrists offices were filled with people who were 'more human than neurotic'. It was a minority who needed the psychiatrist's surgery.[5]

She avoided pathologising 'nerves' by giving people labels for their nervous ailments and did not like to identify 'agoraphobia or other fears by their technical names because she believed labelling a patient's illness does more harm than good',[6] *The San Francisco Examiner* reported in 1969 in an article titled 'Learn How Not to Fight Fear'.

Many headlines invoked the housewife, although Weekes always identified men as equally susceptible. Some refused promotions. Powerful men also panicked. 'Tycoons walk three flights up to avoid getting into an elevator; board chairmen drive 30 miles so they won't have to cross a certain bridge,' she told the *Los Angeles Times*.

The popular talk shows picked her up. She appeared on the ABC in the US, where she was a guest on *The Dick Cavett Show*, at the more serious end of the spectrum. He rated third in the genre, behind Johnny Carson and Merv Griffin. On 14 October 1969, she was interviewed on Griffin's program on CBS, along with Clint Eastwood and Sacha Distel.

Coincidently, 1969 was the year when 'the field of neuroscience was officially born as a discipline', according to Joseph LeDoux, a renowned US neuroscientist himself.[7] With psychoanalysis and behavioural psychology still jostling for pre-eminence, it would be years before a more biological approach would be back in therapeutic favour, ushered in by neuroscience. Weekes, with her emphasis on the nervous system and the concept of first and second fear, anticipated the return to biology and the physiology of the brain decades later.

Her success as an author was replicated in front of a

microphone or a camera, given her ability to simplify and communicate a complicated story about the mind–body connection. When interviewed, she found such an unexpectedly responsive audience that the television networks were willing to pay for expensive accommodation and limousines. Her days of celebrating third-class travel were a memory.

It was easy to measure Weekes' success, as her interviews elicited a more visceral response than the celebrities who had sat in the same chair. The phrase 'melted the switchboard' was a regularly recurring metaphor to describe the effect she had on broadcast audiences, and it was certainly true of her interview on the ABC network with Virginia Graham, whose successful daytime television talk show, *Girl Talk*, attracted roughly two million viewers five days a week. Graham's audience tuned in to listen to interviews with celebrities such as the actors Bette Davis, Lucille Ball, Liza Minnelli, Olivia de Havilland, and Glenda Jackson and the powerful wives of political leaders, such as Dewi Sukarno.

When Graham asked her producer — identified as Monty in her memoirs, *If I Made It, So Can You* — which of her famous guests had drawn the most response, she was told, to her utter astonishment, that it was Dr Claire Weekes. 'She lives in Sydney and she was a remarkable guest. When we had her on, the people would call during commercials crying, "where can I reach that doctor?"' Monty said.

Graham herself did not admit to fear. 'Everybody I have ever leaned on has been a pillar of Jell-O, and I've just never had anybody to turn to. I guess maybe that makes you strong,' she said, and 'I know people who would rather have two weeks at the Mayo Clinic than go to Europe.'[8] Monty, however, was not surprised at the popularity of Weekes, and he never forgot her. Ten years after Weekes appeared on *Girl Talk*, he visited her in Sydney.

In the US, Weekes found the same sort of previously unmet

demand for her nostrums as she found in the UK. People would befriend her and offer hospitality, but it was not all uncomplicated gratitude. Some were captivated by uncharted commercial opportunities and wished to appoint themselves her navigator, while others were so impressed with the power of her work that they just picked it up and turned it into their own product, with or without acknowledgement. Mainly, people just wanted to spread the word in their own communities or organisations.

Back in Australia, the doorbell rang, as well as the phone. Weekes continued to take in needy people, despite a busy life. Some were prepared to travel to Australia to get help. When they got the dedicated Weekes package, some expected a big bill. Weekes' niece Lili remembers the Texan desperate to reward her aunt for curing his wife when he discovered Weekes intended charging him only her normal consultation fee.

'I will never forget this,' Lili says, adopting a Texan accent: 'Dr Weekes, what are you talking about?' Lili laughs, saying Weekes shrugged it off. 'That's what I mean about Aunty, she was just dedicated, and she said: no, no that's my fee.'

Frustrated, the Texan 'went to Gucci and had a special handbag made just for Aunty Claire to put her scripts in, to carry her books when she was travelling,' Lili adds. 'She had a few [patients] like that. She charged a minimal fee and then they gave her presents. One sent a brooch with diamonds on it. She wasn't expecting any of that.'

Generally, the response confirmed Weekes' experience of treating anxiety in her surgery in Sydney. People got better. Once her books were published, letters from readers started, and never stopped. 'In Sydney we used large green plastic garbage bags about a metre deep,' Weekes wrote to Robert DuPont a year before she died, 'and I have crowned one of these with notices about my work, some of them pretty startlingly good.'⁹

Her business dealings were as basic as the large green garbage bags. Sometime in the middle of the 1960s, Weekes indulged her preference for making business partners out of avid admirers who believe they had been cured by her books. They understood passionately the power of her work, and she rated this above any commercial considerations.

She established a relationship with the Texan businessman Jack Yianitsas in 1966. The relationship was to last a decade only to end in confusion, estrangement, and a messy legal battle — first with Weekes herself and then, decades later, with her relatives.

Yianitsas started life as a salesman for office furniture, having originally hoped to work in theatre. He eventually found an outlet for his theatrical instincts by setting up a company, Success Dynamics, which produced self-help recordings. From this platform, Yianitsas gave motivational speeches around the country, yet the man selling confidence had a breakdown himself, admitting himself to hospital emergency departments to treat his severe anxiety attacks.[10]

It was during what he calls a 'dark period in my life' that Yianitsas found *Hope and Help for Your Nerves* in a library, wrongly catalogued in the religion section. The book cured him. Yianitsas became another grateful reader intent on contacting the person who had given him back his life. 'Her methods made such a tremendous impact on my life, my survival and complete total recovery, that I sought out Dr Weekes, to meet and thank her personally.'[11]

Yianitsas received a personal response from Weekes herself, after he had approached her publisher. Before reading her book, he had been seeing more than one psychiatrist and had no idea what was wrong with him, his terror compounded by an income dependent on his ability to address huge, live corporate audiences. Panic attacks and motivational speeches were a hard combination to manage.

For ten years, the doctor and the businessman were tied together personally and professionally. Weekes gave Yianitsas, with his soft voice and Texan warmth, her total trust. He found her 'extremely comfortable to be with', and they talked about 'everything' together. Given his own experience in the self-help genre, Yianitsas saw an opportunity to extend her brand, and the business. Weekes stayed at his home in Texas, along with Coleman, whom Yianitsas describes as 'sweet, gentle, and kind'. He accompanied Weekes on her trips around the US, helping to arrange TV and radio interviews. Weekes' hardback book was out of print when he met her, he says, and he claims it was his own idea to 'plant the seed' with a US publisher to release it in paperback.

By his own account, he then persuaded her to make a series of audio recordings, and the result was *Hope and Help for Your Nerves*; *Good Night — Good Morning*; *Moving to Freedom*; *Going on a Holiday*; and *Freedom from Nervous Suffering*, with Yianitsas the sole distributor.

He counted her, he says, as a friend, and argues that he had no interest in financial gain for himself and that his only purpose was to assist others to obtain her work 'in order to accelerate their recovery from nervous illness'.[12]

It was an unorthodox arrangement. They set up a company called Galahad Productions, which basically consisted of a bank account in Weekes' name. Money for the LP recordings of her work would be posted to Yianitsas, and he would bank it on her behalf, he explains.

Weekes eventually acknowledged she was no businesswoman, and if she started out not knowing this, there were many confirmations of it in the years to come. Money did not interest her enough, and she was personally frugal. Always judicious with her own obligations, she was nonetheless generous with money when it involved friends or family and so she was oblivious to the risks of mixing the professional and the personal, with its inevitable conflicts of interest. There was no one to save her from herself.

Weekes, Yianitsas contends, was a genius. Her faith in him was such, he says, that she appointed him as her proxy in the US, able to provide therapy based on her work, free of charge. Weekes had suggested he do so, he says, to save them the expense of ringing to speak to her in Australia.

Yianitsas claims to have counselled many people over the phone on this basis, saying that he turned down an offer of a 15 per cent interest in the business, and that he helped with the demands from the media. Yet he also acknowledges that he saw an opportunity to make money, while insisting this was far from his main motivation.

The trigger for the dissolution of their partnership was, by Yianitsas' account, the publication of his personal story, which he called *From Panic to Peace*, which detailed how he recovered after reading her book. This was his own product, he says, for his own profit, and he embarked on promoting it, believing Weekes would be 'surprised' and 'pleased' that he had attributed his recovery to her program, thus helping publicise her work. He concedes, however, that he feared that, had he asked her permission, she would have withheld it.

He promoted the audio recording on his own letterhead as '"A Personal Story by Jack Yianitsas": A presentation to help you understand, cope and recover from nervous and emotional stress.' The program description in the marketing did not mention the name of Dr Weekes. Yianitsas believed it was his tale to tell. Weekes saw it quite differently: it involved her work and he had not sought her permission. It was, she believed, a betrayal of trust.

'Dr Weekes could be somewhat controlling — she dominated or controlled her patients and she wanted blind obedience from all of us,' Yianitsas asserts. Lawyers were called in, but Yianitsas said on the two occasions when 'attorneys got involved' he had produced a letter she wrote to him on her usual blue stationery where he had circled one sentence, which said, 'none of all of this would have been possible without you'.

Weekes eventually folded and withdrew from combat. Yianitsas, who continued to supply her resources to people who wanted them, claims he was only doing it for altruistic reasons and for no personal gain.

Some years after her death, and nearly 20 years after they parted ways, he obtained a video made by Weekes in England and began to market it in the US, although it was sold to him specifically for his personal use alone. As a consequence, Yianitsas would end up in another legal battle with Weekes' heirs. Her aunt's vexed business dealings would give Frances headaches for decades.

For Yianitsas, now well into his 80s, there is a bitter residue. He was so close to Weekes that it felt 'like a failed marriage'. In his disappointment, he claims, he wanted to 'revenge' himself in some way and he now accepts he had no entitlement to Weekes' video, for example. His continuing defence is that he wanted to spread the word, and that any money he made from her work was negligible.

'As I now reflect on the past, her acrimony, lack of recognition and appreciation for my unselfish contribution to her success, triggered a feeling and conviction that I had "earned the right" and justification to seek reimbursement for my years of unconditional commitment and effort to further her cause.'

Yet in 1966 any complications from such ill-fitting business/ patient relationships were unimaginable to Weekes, whose profile was steadily rising with her book sales.

Chapter 23

PEACE FROM AGORAPHOBIA

In 1969, Weekes' words of wisdom nestled among those of celebrities. Under the headline 'Prominent Women Quoted' in the *Statesman Journal*, Weekes was quoted alongside Elizabeth Taylor. 'People should learn to go through life not so immaculately. The important thing is to accept what can't be rectified,' said Weekes.[1]

In November that year, she was described as 'the square built, jolly Australian who spent 12 years in the University laboratory before she decided to go after her medical degree ("So I could work with people"). She tosses her cropped iron-grey head of hair … "I have infinite sympathy and infinite patience with these people. And I never give up,"' she told the *Los Angeles Times*.

In 1972, the American edition of her book, *Hope and Help for Your Nerves*, was a bestseller on the west coast of America and top of the list for overall bestseller in the US according to *Publishers Weekly*, a feat that was, she said, 'quite something for an Australian book!'[2]

It was also remarkable because it achieved this top ranking six years after its first publication. By the end of the '60s, the rest of the world was bidding for her work. She was translated into German in 1964, Afrikaans in 1969, and Spanish in 1972, to be followed shortly by Norwegian, Dutch, Japanese, French, Danish, and Swedish editions. (Later, Hungarian, Thai, and Braille versions would add to the list.) It had been condensed by the popular *Reader's Digest* and by the early 1970s sold an estimated 250,000 copies.[3]

Angus & Robertson were delighted. The head of the general publishing division, John Abernethy, cited Weekes' work as one of the three examples that proved Australian books could appeal to an international audience. (The other two were the novelist Thomas Keneally and the tennis writer Paul Metzler.)

The market for anxiety was now all too obvious. The paper-back edition of *Hope and Help for Your Nerves* was followed in 1971 by another contract with the US publisher Hawthorn Books, and now A&R wanted a second book, which they commissioned, and *Peace from Nervous Suffering* was published in 1972 in the US, Canada, the UK, Australia, New Zealand, and all Commonwealth countries.

There was a catch, however. Although the psychiatric and psychological professions were lately alert to the unmet demand in the anxiety market, as they took a closer look they were simul-taneously beginning to refine new categories. What had earlier become popularised as the housebound-housewife syndrome, now had an important new medical name — agoraphobia. The condi-tion was first diagnosed by German neurologist Carl Westphal in 1872, and had been reintroduced by some well-known figures in the industry, like the British psychiatrist Dr Isaac Marks, who specialised in anxiety and would many years later acknowledge Weekes' work.

Statistics were being thrown around. 'It is estimated that in England 100,000 people suffer with this complaint and that in America there are at least 300,000 nervously ill housebound housewives. There are male agoraphobics too, but not as many,' *The Pensacola News Journal* reported in 1969.[4]

The condition was mainly attached to women, although

Weekes understood it was not gender specific. Far more importantly, she did not like using labels. She avoided them, believing they were worse than counterproductive. 'Patients are individuals … and labelling a patient only tends to give him added fears,' Weekes was quoted as saying.[5]

Her patients and readers had recovered without the definitional refinements to come. The terms 'panic attacks', 'obsessive-compulsive disorder' (OCD), 'post-traumatic stress disorder' (PTSD), 'generalised anxiety disorder' (GAD), and 'social-anxiety disorder' (SAD) were not in use, let alone in acronym form. As the years went on, the disorders would become even more finely sliced, until 2017, when there were 23 separate diagnostic categories of anxiety in the fifth edition of the *Diagnostic and Statistical Manual*, up from ten in *DSM-IV*, and four of them completely new.[6]

Weekes was now described by the media as a pioneer — in agoraphobia in particular — even though she had been critical of the labelling trend, preferring a unified approach to the treatment of anxiety. These new labels all dealt with variants of an identical problem: fear of fear. Whether it be fear of the marketplace, of a contaminated sink, or of bridges, boats, or planes, the wellspring was the same, in Weekes' canon.

It took decades for other professionals to agree, and many didn't and still don't. Scholars built reputations around ever more refined categories of anxiety. The anxiety specialist David Barlow argued in 2017 that this trend to splitting had more to do with funding and tenure than science.[7] Neuroscience and a better understanding of neurobiology later validated Weekes' approach to nervous illness: that it was more useful to understand what was common about a variety of anxiety conditions, than what was different.

Yet while Weekes resiled from labelling, the fascination with agoraphobia was increasing her market value and power. She was now almost full-time on the promotional trail and enjoying the luxuries that attended being an in-demand speaker. This was a 'second command promotion tour', according to newspaper reports, given the belated arrival on the bestseller list of her first book.

Now, as well, she had a new book to promote. *Peace from Nervous Suffering* was a reiteration of her first, with more detail for the avid, anxious market. In one respect, however, it represented capitulation. Her resistance to labels in 1969, on the grounds they just frightened people, had collapsed in the face of the public and professional fascination with agoraphobia. Dr Weekes chose to meet the market.

Agoraphobia was saleable, and her publishers were keen to exploit this new opportunity off the back of her successful first book. Weekes wrote to the brief. *Peace from Nervous Suffering*, she explained in her publicity, was aimed at 'a particular fear', agoraphobia. Her book, she proclaimed, was the first 'written by a doctor directly to sufferers from this crippling illness ... Indeed, other than treatises on agoraphobia written for medical journals, or mention of it in books on fears and phobia, this is the first book written mainly on agoraphobia itself.'

There were other, subtler pressures on her to 'label'. Her friend Joyce Skene Keating was identified as an agoraphobic, and the Open Door, where they first met, was a charity for agoraphobics and actively promoted Weekes' work. Resistance was becoming counterproductive. Weekes wrote *Peace from Nervous Suffering* from Skene Keating's house in London, and, later in life, she pointed out to Bob DuPont that she had stayed with her for 25 years. 'If you really want to know about agoraphobia, live with one [who suffers from it], as often and for as long as I did,' she wrote.

Skene Keating was acknowledged in one of Weekes' later books — but as a friend rather than a sufferer. In *Peace from Nervous Suffering*, Weekes more discreetly penned a dedication 'with esteem to the many whose courage has helped to make this book'.

The wave of interest in agoraphobia continued to swell, and Weekes surfed it for the rest of the decade. Her opportunism didn't alter her premise, that this phenomenon, while incapacitating, was just an iteration of the same old problem, fear of fear.

Therefore, there was a paradox at the centre of her new work. Her analysis and treatment of agoraphobia were indistinguishable from her general approach to nervous illness. Agoraphobia was not a fear of wide-open spaces, or crowds, or leaving one's home. Weekes explained it was the fear of the overwhelming fearful *feelings* that were associated with leaving the safety of home. The problem was inside, not outside. 'Agoraphobics are not afraid of a specific thing. They are afraid of what is inside themselves. They have to learn how to panic without panicking.'

Weekes again battled the stereotype that only women suffered. Her first chapter gave equal billing to trapped men and women: 'The Housebound Housewife, the Citybound Executive'. Weekes acknowledged under a subhead — 'Woman rather than man' — that more women than men suffered from agoraphobia but explained this as a cultural rather than a gender phenomenon, asserting 'a woman's life at home lends itself to the development of agoraphobia'.

Another subhead made her point directly: 'His wife went everywhere with him.' Symptoms were no respecter of sex. Weekes pointed out that 'a nervously ill man complains of the same symptoms as a nervous woman ... The symptoms are not as "feminine" as one has been conditioned to think. Many a deputy chief would be chief today were he not afraid of the travelling involved by seniority. I call this the citybound executives' syndrome.'[8]

She gave it a go, but 'citybound executives' syndrome' did not catch on. Agoraphobia did, and Weekes continued to leverage the condition to get attention. On 27 April 1972, the *Los Angeles Times* reported that 'Dr Weekes, a youthful 70 year old with a cheery, charming manner, paused at the Century Plaza to kick off a nation-wide tour on behalf of the book, *Peace from Nervous Suffering*.'[9] Publicity fed on itself, and she was interviewed again on many of the big networked US radio and TV talk shows, by popular hosts such as Mike Douglas, Arlene Francis, and Barry Farber. On the Mike Douglas show on 26 May, she shared the limelight with Tom Tryon, the Charlie Byrd Trio, and a Roller Games demonstration.

The reviews in the UK were favourable as usual, and the *Guardian* newspaper reviewer called *Peace from Nervous Suffering* a 'marvellously helpful book'.

> In it Dr Weekes explains fully and yet simply each of the myriad symptoms an agoraphobiac may suffer from and puts it all into perspective. She describes the three pitfalls that lead to nervous illness — sensitisation, bewilder-ment and fear. Dr Weekes' previous book *Self Help For Your Nerves* is frequently carried around by agoraphobi-acs who regard it as their Bible. The new work is even more valuable, and until the medical profession does come up with some better answers to this heartrending problem the housebound agoraphobiac could find him or herself getting farther and farther afield by following Dr Weekes's advice.[10]

It was true that many of Weekes' most dramatic success sto-ries had come from treating so called agoraphobics via what she called her 'remote direction' — that is, her books and her audio recordings. If she had agreed with labels, this would be her killer category, as whatever value her work had for anxiety in general, the most evidently remarkable cures were with those people who had been homebound for months, years, and sometimes more than a decade. This amplified her fame as these cases were often regarded as the most intractable.

Peace from Nervous Suffering with its focus on agoraphobia also invited new professional attention. She was asked to write for the *British Medical Journal*, and her article, 'A Practical Treatment of Agoraphobia', was published in May 1973. Weekes used the opportunity to present some statistics to support her claims for successful treatment of this difficult condition.

Throughout the '60s, her years of contact with British self-help groups meant she had access to many so-called agoraphobics who had been using her book and her audio resources. She told *The Sunday Times* in 1973 that she had 2000 patients she had never met.[11] As a result, she had a sizeable cohort she could interrogate via questionnaire to assess the value of her 'remote direction'. She was eager to demonstrate that treatment by book or cassette could work. When 528 agoraphobics in Great Britain and Ireland agreed to participate, she used the data to support her article for the *BMJ*.

The agoraphobics in her survey had been treated for a period of between a few months to six years, and, of these, 60 per cent had been agoraphobic for ten years or more and 27 per cent for 20 years or more, so that most 'could be classed as chronic agoraphobiacs'.[12] Previous treatment had included almost every known orthodox method.

Her conclusion was that 'of the patients aged 14–29, the result was satisfactory to good in 73%; of those aged 30–39 similar good results were found in 67%, and in those aged 40–49 in 55% of patients. Of the older and therefore more difficult group aged 50–74, good progress was made by 49%.'

This article for a professional publication set her up for her next book, which would be specifically directed at the, to date, elusive professional market. Expertise in agoraphobia sounded more impressive than commonsense advice on nerves.

Meanwhile, Weekes continued to juggle radio, television, and newspapers. She was on *Living Easy*, a television program hosted by Dr Joyce Brothers, whom *The Washington Post* called 'the face of American Psychology'.

Ann Landers, one of the most widely syndicated newspaper columnists, with a popular advice column published in 1200 newspapers, gave Weekes' books an ongoing marquee, from the mid-70s on, even though it was 'rare' for her to do book plugs.[13]

Landers published innumerable letters in praise of Weekes' work. As one anonymous but grateful advocate wrote: 'Dr Claire Weekes changed my life. I felt like a new person. You did for me what no doctor could do and I WENT TO SEVERAL. Please, Ann, recommend it again. — Elated In Evanston'[14]

For decades, Landers continued to advocate Weekes' books, and, in 1985, she wrote that 'many years ago I suggested two books by Dr Claire Weekes. Thousands of people wrote to tell me these books cured them of agoraphobia, even though many did not even know the name of the illness. Dr Weekes was the first person, to my knowledge, to write about this illness.'

Weekes' approach was that the dreaded bridge should be crossed, but in a special way, her way, with total acceptance and an understanding of the way in which memory had conspired with the nervous system to keep the body trigger-happy and ready to fire. This was exposure therapy for sure, but on very exact terms. By learning to walk with fear, the individual learned how to walk without it, as Weekes would say.

> You're under stress. Nature answers with a shot of adrenaline. This shot travels like lightning: to the head, the heart, the stomach. You gasp for breath, feel faint, struggle with a sense of nausea, feel a band of iron around your forehead.

Whatever happens, it panics you. The perfectly natural fear that it may happen again tenses you more. And so it does happen again — and a double shot of adrenaline courses right down that original route again. Just as you can wear a path across a vacant lot, if you step on it often enough, your nerves — responding to anxiety and stress and charged on with super doses of adrenaline — set up a freeway route. You're sensitised.

By 1973, Weekes was increasingly publicly critical about psychoanalysis. 'Finding a childhood cause for present illness may be interesting, but it rarely helps cope with the present condition.'[15] People wanted 'urgent relief now. People want to be told what to do — and now. They don't need to be taken back to their childhood and told their mothers didn't love them.'[16] Whatever caused the sensitisation was immaterial. 'The habit of fear is the important thing now. *This must be cured.*'[17]

In those four words, 'the habit of fear', lay scholarship that straddled over a century of work on evolution and the nervous system. Beside this idea was an even more refined and important concept. Weekes explained the difference between what she called 'first and second fear'. Understanding this and then knowing how to manage the difference was at the heart of her work. Her latest book offered an analysis that would anticipate scholarship decades later, of emotions and the brain and the misunderstood phenomenon of fear.

Chapter 24

A PIONEER OF FEAR

'Evolution does the thinking.'

JOSEPH LEDOUX[1]

Joseph LeDoux blames himself for helping create a myth about fear in the brain. The eminent neuroscientist from New York University, celebrated as a 'true leader in the cutting-edge field of neuroscience and psychology',[2] has made a specialty of fear, as well as the 'survival circuits' in the brain that were so important to the work of Weekes.

'The amygdala has become famous as being the brain's fear centre, and I am partly responsible for that ... it has almost become a cultural meme, so it is hard to get past this sort of confusion that a lot of scientists have,' he said in an interview for the Smithsonian Associates program. He has struggled to be heard, even by other scientists. The misconception rules.

Contrary to popular opinion, fear does not 'live' in the brain in a dwelling called the amygdala, LeDoux explains. There are no 'homes' there for thoughts and feelings but instead there are systems, networks, and processes. This clarification of what he means underpins his point that scientific confusion about fear has impeded improved treatment of anxiety conditions. In his 2015 book, *Anxious: using the brain to understand and treat fear and anxiety*, LeDoux argues that fear is so loosely defined that it creates a fog of misunderstanding.

Not only is there not one 'home' of fear in the brain, but there are two quite separate brain systems implicated in the human experience of this emotion. LeDoux makes a crucial distinction between the system that detects and responds to threats — the fight, flight, or freeze mechanism, which he calls the survival circuit where 'evolution does the thinking' — and the system that generates 'conscious feelings of fear'. They operate quite differently.[3]

Weekes would have been in furious agreement as her work was built on a similar premise. While LeDoux refers to a 'two-systems approach', she used popular language and identified 'first and second fear'.

The difference between one and two is vital. LeDoux argues that the failure to distinguish between the two systems has 'impeded progress in understanding fear and anxiety disorders and hindered attempts to develop more effective pharmaceutical and psychological treatments'.[4] In short, pharmaceutical interventions such as antidepressants were based on treating rats' survival circuitry, their fight, flight, or freeze instinct, or what Weekes called first fear. Both LeDoux and psychologist Lisa Feldman Barrett, author of *How Emotions Are Made: the secret life of the brain*, assert that this innate survival instinct is not a mental state at all and should not even be classified as 'fear'.

Although Weekes constantly used the word 'fear', she specifically nominated two very different brain states, and it was this distinction that supported her analysis and her treatment protocol. In her second book, *Peace from Nervous Suffering*, she expanded on her earlier explanation of the nervous system and these two different fears in particular. Understanding how and why they were so different was, she argued, the key to breaking the devastating panic cycle.

Weekes, like LeDoux and Barrett, did not regard first fear as a mental state, being beyond conscious control, and all three have used animal analogies to underline the point, demonstrating how this automatic defence system worked. Weekes wrote pages on the autonomic nervous system, and its two branches, the sympathetic and the parasympathetic, as well as the fear-adrenaline-fear cycle. Fight or flight is a survival circuit, as any evolutionist would know, and is common to all animals — the lizard brain, in popular shorthand. This older brain is indispensable in a genuine emergency, but, when it becomes chronic, activating even when there's no real emergency, it's just destructive. To explain its felt effect on the body, Weekes described it as a 'flash'.

Her 'first fear' was easy enough to identify as the survival response, the dumb alarm of fight or flight. It was 'second fear' that presented more of a challenge to describe. What was it?

Under another reader-friendly headline, 'First Fear Must Always Die Down', Weekes asserted that the whiplash of first fear was followed by a second fear, which she identified as a feeling that could be described as 'What if (add in catastrophic thought)'. First fear launched an orchestra of bodily responses to a perceived threat; and to the pounding heart, the churning stomach, the trembling body was added second fear. 'Oh my goodness here it is! I can't stand it. I might make a fool of myself in front of all these people! Let me out of here! Quickly. Quickly. Quickly.'

Although she did not give it a neurological definition, her 'second fear' invoked another brain process in human beings — that of conscious emotion, which involved a different matrix in the brain, or what LeDoux later called 'cortical consciousness networks',[5] a more-recent evolutionary development. These networks (rather than the more popular notion of the prefrontal cortex) gave rise to consciousness, which allowed for reflection, thought, self-consciousness, and anxiety.

The first fear that Weekes identified took the fast road and manifested itself in less than the blink of an eye. The second fear, which consciously reflected on the first and was a fearful appraisal of it, was infinitesimally slower. Weekes identified the treacherous collaboration between the two that delivered the vicious cycle of panic. The first fear, she said, was 'normal in intensity; we understand it and accept it because we know that when the danger passes, the fear will also pass'. However, in the case of a sensitised person, that flash of first fear can be 'so electric in its swiftness, so out of proportion to the danger causing it, that he cannot readily dismiss it. Indeed, he usually recoils from it, and as he recoils he adds a second flash of fear. He adds fear of the first fear. Indeed, he may be much more concerned with the physical feeling of panic than with the original danger. And because that old bogie, sensitisation, prolongs the first flash the second flash may seem to join it. This is why the two fears feel as one.'

LeDoux years later concluded that 'threat processing contributes to maladaptive feelings of fear and anxiety', and that people who suffer from fear and anxiety disorders are 'hypersensitive to threats' and become hypervigilant.

Weekes 'acceptance' protocol was designed to short-circuit the fear cycle that was launched by sensitisation or hypervigilance. It also assumed that the more modern part of the brain, its reasoning system, could not override the more primitive survival circuits of fight and flight.

Therefore, to achieve 'peace from nervous suffering', the body, not just the mind, needed to be engaged, and this was the point of her treatment mantra of 'facing, accepting, floating, and letting time pass'. It downregulated the nervous system so that second fear would not recharge the dumb alarm of first fear, offering the possibility of handing power back to the sufferer. Fighting fear was as useless as the sufferer trying to 'think' their way out of the problem by employing the frontal neocortical connections, which have no control over these primal survival circuits. Indeed, the neuroscience has shown exactly the opposite: thinking is impeded in the panic state. Reason is not transcendent, a point made even earlier by Carl Jung:

> A fundamental principle of my work is that any developmental theory must integrate psychology and biology. For the last two decades, I have argued that no theory of human functioning can be restricted to only a description of psychological processes; it must also be consonant with what we now know about biological structural brain development.[6]

LeDoux explains the different processes this way:

> if you have a brain that can be conscious of its own activities you can become aware that when this brain system is activated that you see yourself freezing and notice that your heart is beating fast, that you are experiencing a state of fear. And that is a conscious experience. That is not bubbling up out of the amygdala but that is being actively assembled in the higher centres of the brain, in the cortex, particularly the pre-frontal cortex by that kind of knowledge or understanding of the situation you are in. So, it is a completely different thing and it is possibly something that is uniquely human.[7]

Here would be Weekes' idea of second fear.

Weekes also pointed out the fierce tenacity of brain habits, entrenched by memory, to which the body responded reflexively. Such habits must be broken. Weekes argued this was achieved by acceptance or, by *not* adding second fear to first. As she would say countless times, 'simple but not easy'. The nervous system had been trained to respond in a negative circuit and instead had to learn to 'panic without panicking'. The objective, she counselled, was that these bodily responses 'no longer matter'.

Barrett puts it this way: 'your body primes your mood'.[8] Like many others, she turned to neuroscience to understand emotional life, and she argues that emotions are not things that happen to us but are constructions we make.

In Barrett's view, 'everything you feel is based on a prediction of how you feel from your knowledge and past experience. You are truly an architect of your own experience. Believing is feeling.' Along with LeDoux, she regards fear as a more complex state than fight, flight, or freeze. Rather, a group of 'interoceptive networks' in the body 'predict' the future, thus forming the basis of emotions. For example, the heart races when a critical boss approaches although there are no plans to run. The prediction could become automatic, triggering the nervous system into action.

If your brain constantly uses past experience, as Barrett argues, and changes your mood, then Weekes was attempting, via acceptance, to keep the power of memory in check, as the brain and body could be primed by sensitisation to hold fiercely to the memory of those surges of uncontrollable fear and so began to anticipate them far too readily.

Although acceptance, or not fighting, lay at the centre of her treatment, Weekes had some other novel techniques, one of which she called 'glimpsing', or finding a new point of view. Glimpsing was a technique to manage some difficult problem that was perpetuating anxiety. To begin with, Weekes said, the individual, possibly with help, needed to find a less painful way of looking at the situation. 'He must find a new point of view.'

> If he can glimpse the new point of view for a few moments each day he would have made a beginning. Indeed, this is the beginning. Although he may repeatedly lose that glimpse and often despair, if you persevere the glimpse will gradually grow clearer, steadier, last longer, until it becomes established compromise to bring peace at last.[9]

In other words, break the cycle of memory, 'the habit of fear'. Weekes used this technique particularly with patients suffering from obsessions.

Martin Seif, a New York clinical psychologist and founding member of the Anxiety and Depression Association of America, knew Weekes and her work well. 'The real reason old-timers like me keep on invoking Claire Weekes is we actually use the terms first fear and second fear. What is amazing about it is that her description fits the neurology, which was discovered later.'

In his book *Behave*, the neurobiologist and primatologist Robert Sapolsky concludes that the possibilities for neuroplasticity in the brain are 'exciting and promising' but often limited — with one important exception. He thinks the benefits are mostly 'psychological'.[10] Weekes anticipated such neuroplasticity in the brain, at least in relation to mood, and her simple method was designed to lower the sensitisation she blamed for so much bewildering arousal of distressing feelings of fear.

Towards the end of his scholarly tome on anxiety, LeDoux concludes that meditation may be one method of moving into a state that short-circuits the cognitive construction of feelings of fear or anxiety.[11] This is another form of acceptance, although Weekes preferred her version of floating past to staying still.

Chapter 25

LIVING IN TWO WORLDS

In the early 1970s, Weekes and Coleman planned a longer a trip abroad. Dulcie's three daughters were now married and, as Dulcie was living alone, a decision was made to move her upstairs into Weekes and Coleman's apartment, leaving downstairs free for short-term rentals. The first tenants were an American dietician and her husband, who stayed for six months. The second lessee was the famous Australian current-affairs host Michael Willesee, young and newly single, whose time in the apartment saw a host of visiting celebrities, including feminist icon Germaine Greer.

Eventually, Weekes and Coleman returned from overseas. The latter had become even more passionately interested in cooking, and intently watched Robert Carrier's television show, experimenting with his rich European cuisine. It was not long before she reached the limits of the Weekes digestive system with meals infused with wine, garlic, and spices.

Weekes preferred simple food, regarding it as fuel, although she loved a cake. Caraway seed was a favourite, according to Frances. Her aunt could be fussy. She had eaten garlic in France 30 years ago and still didn't like it. Coleman was encouraged to bake instead, and so cakes, biscuits, and pastries became her fallback culinary passion.

Home again, Weekes missed travel, and the big life that went with it. 'When she started making the money from the books, she went everywhere first class, and she was used to everything being first class. She would travel on the Concorde,' recalls her niece Lili.

Beyond the perks of overseas travel, Weekes lacked intellectual stimulation in Australia. She loved her immediate family, but they had little in common. Then there were the dramas. 'When she came back, she was very unsettled.' It was home, but, as Lili points out, 'Home bought lots of problems.'

He wasn't at the top of the list of her family problems, but her brother could be tiring. 'Oh God, it's Brian,' Lili remembers her saying at one of his regular visits. Weekes herself could be self-absorbed, and her work came first, but she was the matriarch, and members of the family turned to her from time to time to solve their problems. She was, however, soon to be delivered a suite of her own.

Tita separated from her husband and moved to a nearby boarding house with her two boys. Feeling this was far from ideal, Weekes and Dulcie conspired to draw her back with them. Weekes wanted Tita, whom she dearly loved, living downstairs. If there was one of her nieces she regarded as a daughter, it was Dulcie's youngest. Tita had been only seven when her father left, and her mother had fallen apart in the aftermath. Weekes was protective of this young girl in whom she recognised emotional vulnerability, yet this relationship, so close to Weekes' heart, would be torrid as well as tender. Tita was pretty, intelligent, volatile, and fragile. The depth of Weekes' feelings and her sense of Tita's fragility was captured in a letter she wrote to her adult niece.

'Knowing you, you will suffer very much. You were born with your heart exposed and an arrow pointed right at it,' Weekes wrote to a young woman whose potential she recognised, and whom she had tried to encourage into employment. 'I don't want you worried — I want you to have a clear brain for your work because that's where your future lies. All you've been through was a life's university course and you passed that with honours.'

Having returned to Cremorne, with her sons, Tita was to turn into a helpmeet, a confidant, a carer, a patient, and occasionally a combatant. It was a mixed experience for both women. Each believed they understood the other, although this did not guarantee harmony. It was Tita's view that her aunt had trained herself to be calm and needed to practise this as she was so easily aroused.

She acknowledges the same was true of herself. 'She only had to look at me to know what I was feeling. She would tell me what I was seeing, and I would say I don't want to go there. She knew me because she knew herself and was not unlike me.'

Weekes tended to assume she could get involved in very personal aspects of Tita's life, and did. Tita felt her aunt attempted to control those she loved. Her aunt's advice was always right, Tita concedes, but she chafed at the oversight and lack of privacy, and could lash out.

Impatient with her aunt's impeccable restraint, Tita made efforts to break it. She was rewarded once, delighted to have provoked Weekes into losing her temper. 'I laughed I was so glad. I said, "Oh good, you can lose your temper." Because I think it's important to get it all out.'

Weekes meted out the same medical treatment to her niece as she gave Dulcie, prescribing sedatives. Again, this was not met with the unanimous approval of this family of noticers, but Dr Weekes was never challenged.

Tita's return to 37 Milson Road brought another generation under Weekes' large umbrella. Adam and Jason were three and six years old, respectively, when their mother returned to her family home. They were raised to understand there were rules upstairs, the most important of which was 'Don't bother Aunty'. But Adam squeezed past Coleman's Praetorian Guard with a mix of charm and compliance. The preschooler was welcome upstairs once he demonstrated that he understood the two women liked things done in a particular way. He knew he had to ring the doorbell, and manners had to be observed. He soon inveigled his way into their breakfast routine.

'It felt like a formal occasion every morning, and I was allowed to join in, which was very special. It was always eggs on toast and a cup of tea, and I was young, and I would have a cup of water or whatever. They were very British, very traditional, and everything with silver service.'

The ritual continued for years. 'They were very particular about table settings and etiquette. They taught me manners.' Adam learned how to hold his knife, and his great aunt would correct his diction. Weekes 'was changing the world', Adam understood, and it was important to fall in line. All her media triumphs were celebrated, and the mail never stopped, which suited a young stamp collector. They watched tennis together every summer, a sport his aunt followed passionately. Another favourite broadcast was the game show *Sale of the Century*.

It wasn't just his aunt who had his affections, as, for the first time, Coleman found a Weekes other than Claire to openly love, and Adam was ready to receive and return it. He was also deeply attached to his 'wonderful' grandmother Dulcie, whom he turned to when his mother was troubled. The breakup with her husband, and the responsibility for two children had compounded the problems for the already 'nervy' young woman.

Weekes saw how stressed Tita could become, and she made efforts to steady her niece. She read Tita's moods. 'She practised on me. She did! She used to see me in a state, and she said, "Just sit down and calm down," and she helped me. All you had to hear was that voice,' said Tita. 'We are a highly strung family — she said we were a family of racehorses.'

All her nieces took their problems to Aunty. The boys learned to follow. Adam remembers that his own father thought Weekes 'hated men'. Yet this was so obviously not true of Lili's husband, Nigel, whom Weekes adored.

Weekes valued her role as family doctor. Tita understood this and once, in an act of rebellion, consulted another doctor over her digestive problem. She knew her aunt would take it badly, and she did. Hurt and furious as she was, Weekes could not resist asking Tita what this new medical rival had prescribed. When she finally extracted the information, she was derisive, telling Tita she had been given the wrong treatment.

Increasingly, Weekes was living in two separate worlds. While her immediate family understood her international fame, she was still an aunt and a sister. Abroad, Weekes attracted women who loved her like an aunt or a mother but revered her as well.

By 1976, the US publishers boasted that *Hope and Help for Your Nerves* 'had been endorsed by medical and medical health professionals throughout the world. Millions of Americans heard Dr Weekes on television and radio and had read excerpts of her book which appeared in Reader's Digest.'[1] Nevertheless, broad professional recognition remained beyond reach.

Weekes was struggling to control Yianitsas and his marketing of her work in the United States when yet another lay fan came knocking on her door. A Florida-based businessman named Steven Reich flew to Australia to meet her, then became a regular visitor. He was a troubled man in his early 30s with a failed marriage, and had been in and out of hospital by the time he discovered Weekes.

In Reich, she found another gratifying acolyte. He also saw a genius and — dazzled as he was — an opportunity. Weekes succumbed to his assiduous attentions, allowing Reich to stay in her home in Australia. At first, he seemed a stalwart. When he wasn't in Australia, he kept in touch by phone. Weekes introduced him to Yianitsas, who later claimed Reich was one of the many Americans he counselled on her behalf to ostensibly save them the cost of phone calls to Australia. Yianitsas claimed that Reich, at one stage, was calling him every day, and that he provided therapy for no charge.

This threesome soon unravelled. When Weekes fell out with Yianitsas in 1977 and needed legal advice, Reich grabbed the chance to become her business partner instead. He recommended his own lawyers, and Weekes swapped one unsatisfactory business arrangement with another that proved to be even worse. According to Yianitsas, Reich subsequently turned up on his doorstep to see if he was continuing to distribute Weekes' work. Reich was to make a habit of these ominous visits to people he viewed as his rivals for her work. Weekes' commercial relationships were about to become even more vexed.

On 18 October 1977, a contract for Worth Productions was drawn up between Weekes, her sister Dulcie, and Steven Reich. He would be the sole distributor of her published audiotapes in the US. Weekes assigned 50 per cent of the royalty rights to Dulcie. They would trade under the name of Galahad Productions, the same name Weekes had shared with Yianitsas. Reich became the general manager of the company and although not paid a salary was entitled to 50 per cent of their net profits.

Reich was a difficult, complicated man. He claimed copyright in the US over any of her audio or video recordings, and the contractual arrangement she had negotiated with him locked out other potentially effective business partners. In front of Weekes, Reich restrained his temper, but others saw a different side.

Until he mysteriously pulled back from contact with Weekes, he visited Australia regularly, staying in her home. When she tired of having him upstairs, she shuffled him downstairs, to Tita's annoyance as she had to make room for him with her mother and two sons. She remembers a tall, slim man, prone to stormy moods. One day, climbing onto a ferry with her and the boys, and furious that he had tripped over the rope on the gangplank, he raged at them.

Tita's sons simply regarded Reich as another one of the 'odd' people their great-aunt had staying with her. But they were impressed by the fact that he was, apparently, a millionaire, and saw an opportunity for themselves. Reich might have been just the sponsor they needed to secure the BMX bikes they yearned for. To their chagrin, they ended up with sweatshirts instead.

Over the years, Reich became unmanageable. He seemed to be sitting on the audiotapes instead of selling them. Weekes was increasingly frustrated as he became elusive, and she worried that openings were being missed to promote her work. Like Yianitsas, Reich would disappoint, but this relationship cut much deeper. Weekes tolerated far more from Reich than anyone else. He may have been convinced that she could cure anyone of nervous illness, yet she never achieved unambiguous success with him. So Weekes had what she would call Reich's 'illness' to contend with, but this already complicated relationship would be further burdened. She would eventually grow frightened of him.

That was all ahead. Now all she saw was a glittering potential in Reich. She was seduced by his intense blandishments. The year 1977, which had opened with such expectation, would end with a personal tragedy, marking the beginning of her turbulent last decade.

Chapter 26

THE SOULMATE

Weekes' third book, *Simple, Effective Treatment of Agoraphobia*, was launched in 1977, a decade and a half after she first burst into print. This was a chance to step from the noisy acclaim of the popular market into the more sedate reception of the professional auditorium, from where a permanent place in history was more likely to be assured.

The 'self-help' noose that had choked off recognition for Weekes was loosening as the media now described her as a 'pioneer' or an 'expert', and occasionally quoted her in the company of other serious professionals, such as the man who would later that year savage her publicly, Dr Joseph Wolpe.[1]

By now, over 300,000 copies of *Self Help for Your Nerves* and the US version, *Hope and Help for Your Nerves*, had been sold in hardback alone. Her second book, *Peace from Nervous Suffering*, had sold 50,000 copies. Six thousand albums of two long-playing records on nervous illness had been purchased in Britain, the United States, and Canada, among other countries.[2] Defying the usual shorter sales cycle of self-help books, Weekes' work seemed evergreen after 15 years.

Angus & Robertson held the rights to *Simple, Effective Treatment of Agoraphobia* in the Commonwealth of Nations, and Hawthorn Books held them in North America. There were varying estimates of the numbers of sufferers floating about, and Hawthorn claimed that there were more than one million Americans with the condition. The US press introduced Weekes as one of the first to talk publicly about agoraphobia. To give her latest book on agoraphobia a scholarly flavour and to support her claim to successful treatment, she based the book on 'facts', referring to her survey of 528 agoraphobic men and women in the UK, 'whom I had treated for periods ranging from one to seven years'.[3]

In her introduction, she offered some jaunty advice to the late 'Dr Freud', who had acknowledged that psychoanalysis had failed to help some of his patients. 'He was dejected when he saw them leave his care still ill,' she wrote. 'Perhaps, had he used a different approach to these people — even such as are described in this book and which differs fundamentally from psychoanalysis — he may have been more successful with them.'[4]

Weekes' own approach remained unchanged. She had capitulated to the label but had not changed her mind that it was just another example of 'fear of fear', that the problem was inside not outside, despite its denomination. Had she been able to see into the future, she would have enjoyed the vindication. Over 30 years after *Simple, Effective Treatment of Agoraphobia* was published, the pre-eminent anxiety specialist Dr David Barlow confirmed what she knew, that the problem was inside not outside.

'We discovered mostly in the last decade,' he wrote in 2008, 'that one of the major difficulties with people with all emotional disorders is that they become very avoidant of their own emotional life. And that panic attacks can be very frightening experiences. So, we are now at the point where we almost come full circle, we still use our exposure techniques, but the actual context of the exposure is often dealing with individual internal emotional life.'[5]

Barlow had come to understand that exposure would not work on its own, as it was the internal feelings or emotions that needed to be accepted and addressed before the agora, or any other fear, could be managed. He acknowledged that agoraphobics' distress was driven by 'the intense negative emotion itself. That's where we think the action is.'[6]

Simple, Effective Treatment of Agoraphobia was the book where Weekes explicitly acknowledged that panic could return, and that her idea of a cure was that this was 'an almost inevitable part of recovery'. Thus she emphasised 'the necessity of learning how to cope with panic itself, and not trying to get used to a feared situation. Recovery means being able to cope with panic and other nerve symptoms and does not necessarily mean the total abolition. How could it, when we must all feel stress and symptoms while we live?'[7]

In January, accompanied as usual by Coleman, Weekes began a two-month, twenty-two-city tour of the United States. On 3 February 1977, Weekes and Dr Manuel Zane (the American psychiatrist who had established the first hospital-based phobia and anxiety clinic in the United States, at White Plains, New York) were guests on NBC's *Tomorrow*, with popular host Tom Snyder, 'the pioneer of late-night television talk shows'.[8] The program ran for 39 minutes and was the most watched program in this timeslot.[9] The next month, she was on the nationally syndicated *Lou Gordon Program*.

Her agoraphobia credentials swelled. The newspaper *Newsday* referred to her as 'one of the world's most widely quoted authorities on the phobia'. Beyond any discourse on agoraphobia, Weekes was offering a different portrait of anxiety in place of the usual picture of neuroticism. She was typically upbeat. Nervous suffering was 'a privilege'. People who had experienced it, she said, were 'more mature, more compassionate than others. Things like music and poetry have deeper meaning for them. I'm sorry for the people who haven't had nervous suffering. A person who has is more interesting than one who hasn't!'

Far from sufferers being neurotic, she asserted that 'it's mostly the racehorses who develop agoraphobia. They are brave, ordinary people and it does them good to be told that.' She cited Dr Isaac Marks, who had remarked that agoraphobics represented a cross-section of the community and were 'not especially neurotic'. This had also been her experience of patients, she said.[10]

Weekes told *The Tennessean* she was 'a real doctor'. She 'had been a researcher but liked working with people. When you have been a doctor as long as I have you respect people. And the feeling of helping them makes it feel worthwhile.'

For the first time since their singing days, Coleman was mentioned in a press report. Yet Weekes' reference to her lifetime soulmate fell well short of respect. Her description of her partner could have been written by her mother, Fan. When *The Tennessean* noted the presence of 'a friend, Miss Elizabeth Coleman', Weekes had 'laughingly introduced "Miss Tagalong" as her travelling companion'.

'Miss Dragalong' might have been more accurate. Coleman found these promotional tours a great strain. With Weekes on her third book, Coleman knew exactly what a coast-to-coast trip entailed. Before the two women left Australia, Coleman had been uncharacteristically distressed at the prospect of the trip, and resistant. She had always put Weekes first, but now she was dreading the long, tiring travel involved in the promotional tours: the hotels, the airports, the long flights.

For the first time anyone could remember such a thing, Coleman was found crying in her room by one of Weekes' nieces. She was 77 years old, her heart was troubling her, and she was tired. Yet Weekes prevailed, and the two women left for the US.

Although the trip did not begin well, Weekes had good reason to anticipate another publishing triumph. She was not to know then that *Simple, Effective Treatment of Agoraphobia* would be a comparative flop. It would be her least saleable book, and, while the others lived on, it was out of print by 1992. At the time, however, it worked well enough to draw an invitation to address an audience of psychiatrists at the 18th Annual Fall Conference of the Association for the Advancement of Psychotherapy, in New York on 23 October 1977, though this, too, would turn out to be a disappointment.

While this first big professional outing was combative and discouraging, public recognition continued to grow. On 7 November, Weekes was quoted at length in *Time* magazine on her theory that agoraphobia was not 'a true phobia. It is one phase of an anxiety state.' Normally, such a mention in a powerful publication would be savoured and reported home.

This was no normal day, however. Weekes was sitting beside an unconscious Coleman in the Mount Sinai Hospital in Los Angeles. At the very end of their trip and just as they were to board a plane home for Sydney, Coleman, who had so expressly resisted more travel, had collapsed on the tarmac at Los Angeles International Airport.

Weekes tried desperately to revive her, without success. An ambulance raced to the hospital, where Coleman hung between life and death for another ten days, never regaining consciousness. She died on 10 November, aged 77; Weekes was a robust 74.

Holding Coleman's hand as she lay in the hospital, Weekes had plenty of time for reflection. The woman whom ten months before she dubbed Miss Tagalong had tagged along for over 40 years. When Weekes wrote in her books about the need to talk about problems, she stressed the importance of picking 'one wise counsellor' — Coleman had been her model, which was confirmed by the sole public homage Weekes paid her lifetime companion, in a dedication in the front of her next book:

... to the memory of Elizabeth Coleman, who always put obligation before inclination and love and loyalty before all else.[11]

Weekes flew back to Australia accompanied by the body, and Coleman's funeral was held in Sydney on 20 November, ten days after her death. Brian and his wife watched Weekes anxiously on the sidelines, fearing the fallout from this unanticipated loss.

The next month, another of Weekes' exceptional success stories was featured in *The New York Times Magazine*. A man known only as 'Peter' had suffered for many years with a kaleidoscope of terrifying symptoms that had left him only able to crawl. He had seen 26 psychiatrists and as many neurologists, taken 32 different drugs — and then, with one phone call to Weekes (he remembered her name from the jacket of a book he was too sick to read), he was cured. He was 'playing tennis' a month later, according to the report.[12]

In its final edition for 1977, *The New York Times Literary Supplement* listed *Peace from Nervous Suffering* at the top of its list of runners-up for sales that year. Usually, this sort of recognition would have given her immense pleasure, but Weekes was in no shape to receive it; glory had been eclipsed by grief.

Apart from the fatigue of bereavement, there were a host of practical issues, including a bill for tens of thousands of dollars for Coleman's treatment at Mount Sinai. For an Australian doctor who charged modest fees or none at all, the American medical system was an unhappy revelation. Amid her own shock and mourning, Weekes found the energy for outrage at the unnecessary medical tests she had witnessed, and the bill that followed. She refused to pay it in full, saying to her relatives, 'Let them sue me.'

She then destroyed her letters from Coleman, and grief took its inevitable path. For a long time, any mention of Coleman's name would bring on tears, and Weekes avoided the bedroom where Coleman had slept. Brian worried about her lack of interest in doing anything at all.

Tita says her aunt was never the same after Coleman's death, although 'she got on with it as she always did'. If one event would test Weekes' own coping abilities, it was this. Weekes had lost her 'soulmate', as Coleman was known by the wider family, and also her daily life, her routine. Coleman had not only offered companionship and intimacy, but run the household. How Weekes could live without Coleman was a very real question.

While they understood the scale of her loss, her family had struggled to understand the relationship between the two women. In their early years together, lifelong female cohabitation was unexceptional and uncontroversial, especially given the surplus of women after the slaughter of World War I. The same was true following World War II, so two women living with family would have attracted little attention until the 1960s burst into being and the next generation enjoyed unprecedented social and sexual freedoms. As time went on, there was speculation within the wider family about the nature of their relationship.

That it was devoted and deep was obvious. What was not so clear was what this meant beyond the bonds of friendship. However intense the interest, no one would have put the question to the protagonists. The relationship was intriguing, but, while occasional discussions ebbed and flowed, they went nowhere, and the women in the wider family accepted the status quo completely.

Paul Skene Keating had been an intimate witness to the relationship between three women: his mother, Weekes, and Coleman. In long conversations with the loving and attentive Coleman, he learned a lot about a woman he knew to be a strict Catholic. He also has a memory of being told that Coleman had been in love with a man, who had broken off the relationship, leaving her devastated. She gave the impression that this was a tragedy that had a deep impact on her life and led to her pulling back from her career as a pianist.

Weekes herself had pulled away, willingly, from her fiancé, Aurousseau. The relationship with Coleman then became the steady and enduring foundation from which she ran her exceptional life.

The two women had shared rooms when they stayed together in Bellevue Hill with Fan and Ralph, but there was no choice in such a crowded house. They had separate bedrooms, as far as anyone knew, once they moved into their own accommodation. Weekes was disinclined to offer physical tenderness, and, in Cremorne, often surrounded by family, the most intimate gesture seen between them was the odd occasion when Weekes would pat Coleman's hand.

It was never entirely relaxing watching the sex scenes on television with Aunty Claire. Her obvious discomfort provoked irritation, amusement, or embarrassment in any niece who happened to be with her when her hands flew to her face, her fingers forming a lattice through which she would peep. For a doctor who had practised medicine for years and claimed to have heard 'everything' about people's secret fears, Weekes remained a square about sex, which she once described quite unromantically and with a biologist's sensibility as 'an itch'.

Only once does anyone recall her discussing homosexuality, in the 1980s. Frances remembers her aunt observing with some sympathy the plight of homosexuals, already so vilified, and suddenly confronting the horror of the newly diagnosed AIDS. 'Now they will be blamed for that, too,' she observed.

Weekes had passion — that much was obvious to anyone listening to her audios or watching her videos, where the intensity of her conviction could be felt. She also had an overactive arousal system, which is why she understood 'nerves' so well. That she

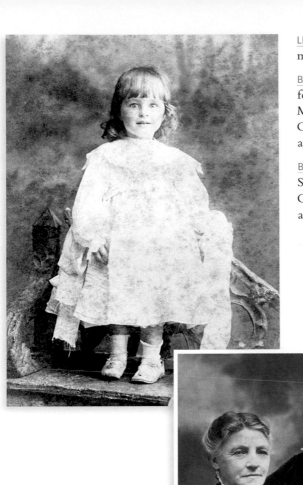

LEFT: Hazel Claire Weekes. Her mother's three-year-old pride and joy.

BELOW: Three generations of formidable Weekes women: Martha Matilda Newland, Claire's grandmother; Claire; and her mother, Fan.

BOTTOM: At home in Bellevue Hill, Sydney, in the 1920s. Brother Brian; Claire; mother, Fan; sister, Dulcie; and father, Ralph.

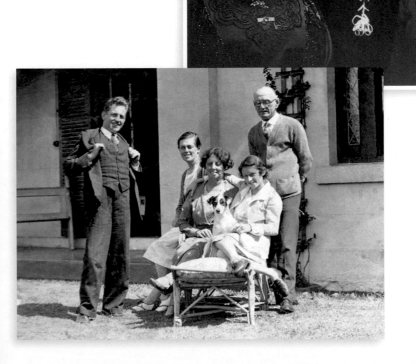

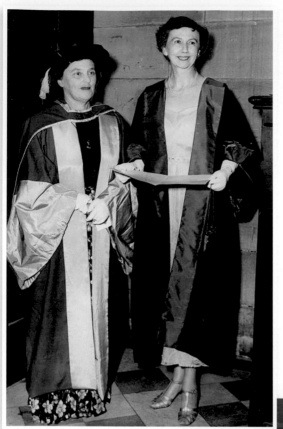

LEFT: The mature-age medical graduate. Dr Weekes is awarded her second degree from the University of Sydney.

BELOW: Thriving in the 1930s, armed with Beth Coleman (right).

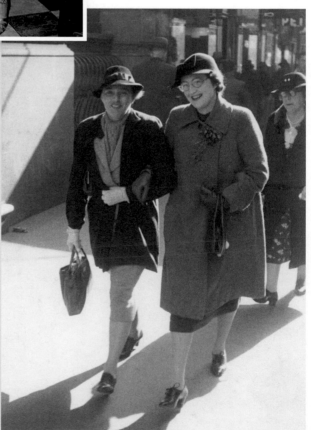

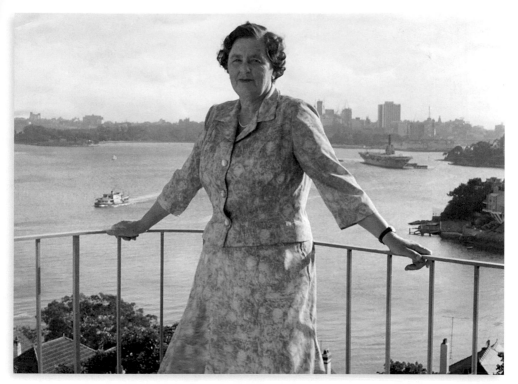

ABOVE: Her great blue view. At home in Cremorne, on the deck overlooking Sydney Harbour.

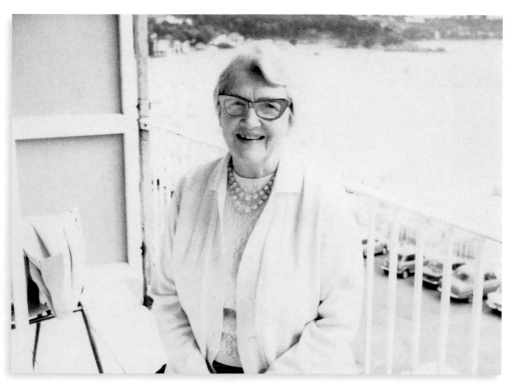

ABOVE: Well travelled. Coleman on one of their many overseas trips.

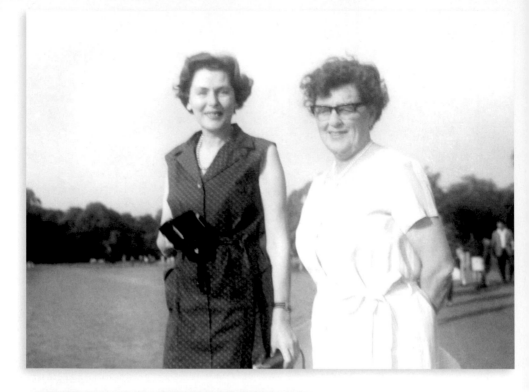

ABOVE: Relaxing with her great friend Joyce Skene Keating (left) in the late 1960s.

LEFT: What an honour. Showing off her MBE. 1979.

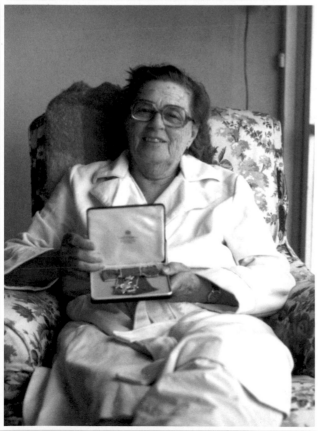

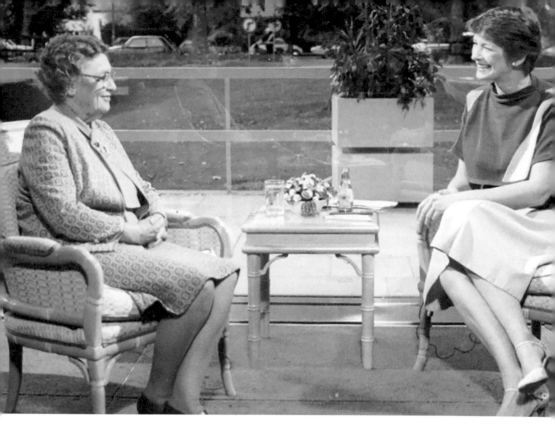

ABOVE: In the limelight with the BBC's Marian Foster in 1983.

BELOW: Happy days. Anne Turner in 1994.

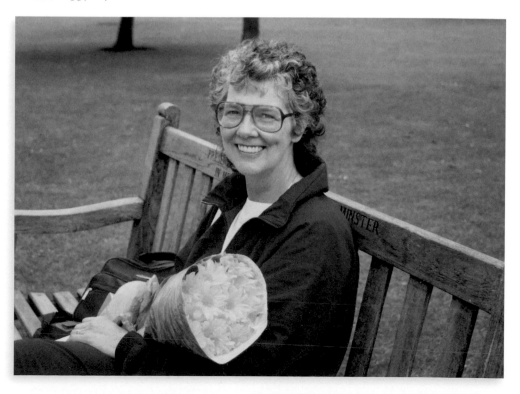

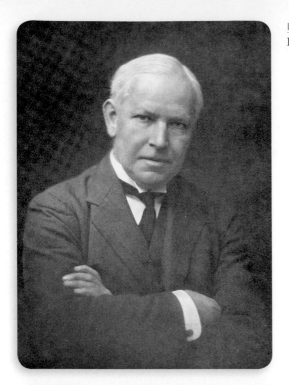

LEFT: The master of the brain, Grafton Elliot Smith. 1920s. *(Wellcome Collection)*

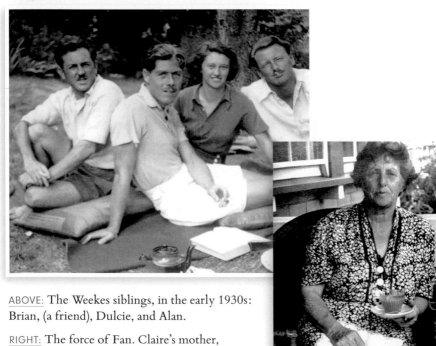

ABOVE: The Weekes siblings, in the early 1930s: Brian, (a friend), Dulcie, and Alan.

RIGHT: The force of Fan. Claire's mother, relaxing with a cup of tea. 1950s.

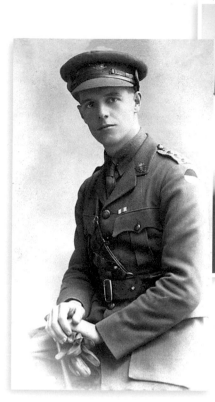

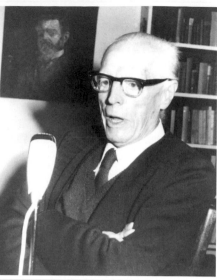

LEFT: Marcel Aurousseau goes to war. 1915.

ABOVE: Marcel Aurousseau, a scholarly old age. 1980s. (*Portrait of Marcel Aurousseau, 30 June 1977 by Hazel de Berg, Courtesy National Library of Australia*)

BELOW: Tender times. Weekes (right), with her niece Tita (centre) and her sister, Dulcie (left).

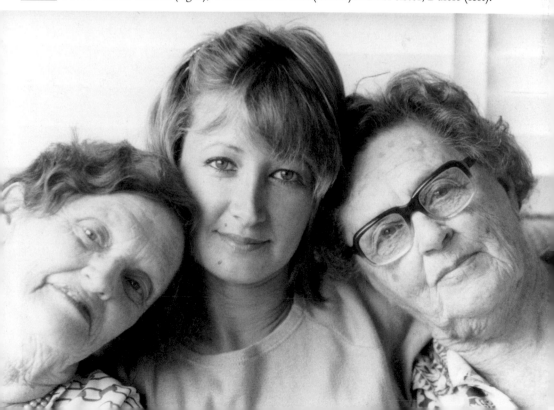

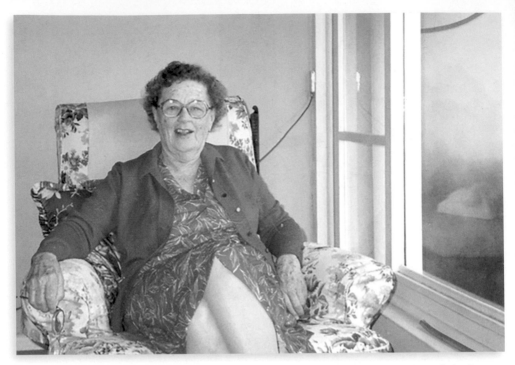

ABOVE: A favourite spot. To her left, the phone that never stopped ringing and a wide harbour view. 1970s.

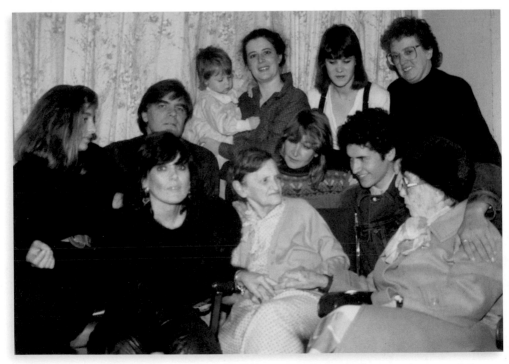

ABOVE: The last year for two sisters. Four generations of Weekeses. (front row) Niece Lili Louez; sister, Dulcie Maclaren; niece Tita Blaiklock; Tita's son Jason; Claire. (back row) Lili's daughter Jacqui Louez; Lili's husband, Nigel Louez; baby Julia Szabo held by her mother, Frances' daughter Josephine Townsend; Frances' daughter Jane Kelly; niece Frances Maclaren.

loved 'Beth' was understood and accepted by all, even slightly envied by those in the family who had been less lucky in romance.

'You know, lovey,' Weekes told Frances in her last years, 'I could never have achieved all this work if I had been married to a man.' Yet while Coleman was alive and doing so much for her, Weekes overlooked the opportunity to publicly acknowledge the woman whose efforts on the home front had helped make it all possible.

She dedicated her first book to her late mother, nominated only nameless anxiety sufferers in her second, and wrote no dedication at all in her third. It was seven years after Coleman had died — in the mid-1980s — that Weekes finally made public what it was that Coleman had meant to her, in the dedication that she wrote in her fourth book. Even there, Coleman huddled in a crowd scene that included other friends and family — but she was the last one on the list of five, and the two words Weekes chose for her were 'love and loyalty'.

Now, without Coleman, Weekes had lost her centre of gravity. The immediate problem was who would pick up all those chores that had fallen to her uncomplaining partner?

It did not take long to see there was a solution at hand: Dulcie. As usual, Weekes got her way. Dulcie, unhappy about leaving her lovely Federation apartment below, was moved upstairs into a more charmless space, leaving her daughter Tita downstairs with her sons.

The compliant Dulcie picked up Coleman's job as homemaker, but she was incapable of providing a *cordon sanitaire* for her sister. There was now no gatekeeper to shut the door, hide behind, vent to, or consult. Weekes was unprotected from the gusty family dramas in a family that rarely underperformed a role.

As the year meandered on, she spent more time with her friends Cecily and Marcel Aurousseau, but she remained grief-stricken, aimless, and restless. Home, even with its prized harbour outlook, had been shrunk by loss.

There were few distractions, and Weekes missed the stimulation of travel and life abroad. She began to resent the tepid professional response to her work, particularly on home ground. Mostly, however, she was adjusting to life without Coleman. In the New Year, she headed to England to be interviewed by BBC radio, and received such a response that she was invited back the following week for a second appearance.[13]

Adrift, Weekes considered her options. There was the pull of Dulcie and the wider family, but they were either absorbed in their own lives or battling their own dramas, which she could find burdensome. Without Coleman, it was tempting to flee to London and move in with a welcoming Joyce Skene Keating and 'Nan' Appleton. Here was another house of women, but without family complications or responsibilities. London, with close friends, offered a closer facsimile of life with Coleman.

One marker of her internal landscape became evident in media interviews. Without her confidant, Coleman, Weekes' professional restraint loosened, and her public comments occasionally included uncharacteristically personal details. In August 1978, she revealed to *The Australian Women's Weekly* for the first time that she herself had suffered from 'the symptoms of stress', and how this had shaped her view that such stress often came on the back of a period of ill health. Perhaps also a sign of her own mood was the disclosure that 'I don't talk about a permanent cure'.[14] This was an important clarification that recovery involved being able to accept and cope with the return of symptoms — a clarification possibly inspired by her own very difficult year. (Five years later, 'cure' was back in her vocabulary, with the caveat that any cure would work only 'as long as the person who has suffered is prepared to live with the memory of that suffering and knows how to cope with its recurrences'.)

The ultimate personal disclosure to *The Australian Women's Weekly*, however, was an announcement that may have surprised her own family. She declared she was thinking of moving permanently to London. What she called her current 'visit' to Australia 'could be her last'. Weekes struck a new critical note about her country and her profession, although it said as much about the missing pieces in her personal life.

She deplored the fact that young doctors did not make home visits, as this, she believed, was where 'real doctoring' was learned. Her main complaint, however, was her local invisibility, given her high profile abroad. Professionals in Australia were not interested in her work. When she spoke about returning to London to live, she added 'it was with regret' that she had received 'no invitation' to tell her colleagues in Australia about her work.

Weekes was chagrined that her work was being 'taught in clinics throughout Britain and America', while in Australia 'only a few therapists are beginning to realise what can be done with my method'. It was this — her work — that was the most important thing in her life. When she referred to her 'work', it was as if it required a capital letter. Always central, it was now an essential stabiliser, as she was unmoored from Coleman. There was more opportunity for her overseas: 'In America I'm dealing with 200 million people, in Britain with more than 50 million.'

Not long after these words were published, Weekes headed to New York, but, in November that year, her brother Alan died suddenly after a heart attack. He was 69 years old. The mysterious pieces of silver paper found in every pocket in Alan's wardrobe after his death turned out to be the antacid Quick-Eze. He had inherited the Weekes gut, but complained to no one of any indigestion, suffering in silence.

The death of her youngest brother, a year after that of Coleman, brought Weekes back to Australia to 'spend Christmas with the family'. There was Alan's funeral to attend, but there was something else drawing Weekes home. She may have been alerted to the forthcoming public acknowledgement she had always yearned for.

In the New Year's Honours list for 1979, Weekes was awarded an imperial honour, an MBE for 'services to medicine'. After a number of her patients had written to the Australian prime minister, Bob Hawke, arguing in favour of her nomination, he had referred the request to the Queen.

The award received modest publicity, and Weekes was forced to carry her own torch in the local media. Her work had greatly influenced psychiatrists around the world, she told *The Australian Women's Weekly*. There had been a change in approach over the past ten to 15 years as they had 'adopted simpler approaches to the treatment of nervous disorders and rejected the Freudian oriented approaches of the past'. The keyword was *simple*. 'The older I get the more value I place on simplicity. Yet simplicity is one of the most difficult things to achieve.'[15]

Chapter 27

VINDICATION

In 1978, a psychiatrist from the Sheppard and Enoch Pratt Hospital, in Baltimore, paid a visit to a colleague in Minnesota. Dr Douglas Hedlund was frustrated with the results he was getting from psychoanalysis in his psychiatric unit at Enoch Pratt, and he had heard that the well-known and respected psychiatrist Dr Arthur Hardy was getting better results with distressed patients by following the methods of an Australian doctor, Claire Weekes. He wanted to know more.

Hedlund returned to Baltimore prepared to try these new ideas of Weekes and to establish an outpatient clinic to treat agoraphobics.

In search of a 'heretic' willing to help him in this endeavour, he found Dr Sally Winston, a Canadian on his staff who had completed a doctorate in psychology from the University of Illinois. Winston was the sole psychologist among all the psychiatrists at the inpatient service in Baltimore and 'was known for my heresy because I was not psychoanalytically trained', she says.

Following the ideas of Weekes was a clear reversal of the usual practice. Psychiatrists — and to an extent, psychologists — followed theorists, not the writers of self-help books. For years, tension shook the leaves on these two different branches of the same tree. Psychiatrists enjoyed a higher status than psychologists because they were trained medical doctors and yet ironically employed very little biological science. They regarded psychologists as less well trained, and, immersed in the mysteries of the unconscious, they bridled against incursions into their terrain.

Such was the popularity and acceptability of psychoanalysis that demand did not inevitably meet supply. Psychiatrists were expensive, too, and there was a gap in the market for psychologists[1] and social workers.

Winston remembers 'the many absurd clinical case discussions' she had heard when working in psychoanalytic hospitals in the 1970s. She was unimpressed with 'how often energy and time was wasted in damaging ways'. She notes that the psychoanalytic treatment seemed inflexible and endless, and anxiety symptoms rarely improved.

'You didn't explain things to people, you didn't answer their questions. What you did was act as a mirror for patients' projections, and you left all the questions hanging because it otherwise invited dependency, and the power of the relationship would be ruined by answering the questions. You didn't talk directly to patients and explain things to them. You just didn't.'

Psychoanalysis was not only ineffective but often had a perverse outcome — some patients got worse rather than better, particularly those patients who suffered from agoraphobic anxiety and obsessive-compulsive disorders, the very people Weekes was treating more successfully.

On the other hand, Winston saw that Weekes worked apparent miracles, having witnessed the remarkable recovery of Zelda Milstein, an intractable agoraphobic who had been cured after reading *Hope and Help for Your Nerves* and *Simple, Effective Treatment of Agoraphobia*.

'Zelda was a wife and mother who had been housebound for about ten years and had been treated by psychodynamically oriented psychotherapy, trying every actual kind of psychotherapy in an effort to get out of the house.' Nothing worked, says Winston, until, somehow, Zelda stumbled across the work of Weekes. Two books, for which she paid a handful of dollars, enabled Zelda to not just overcome her fears but become a paraprofessional therapist herself, under the supervision of Winston, who, like Manuel Zane in New York, was having success with using former sufferers as therapists.

Hardy, Hedlund, and Winston were not alone in their critique of psychoanalysis as the anti-psychiatry movement gained momentum. Thomas Szasz, a Hungarian-born psychiatrist turned anti-psychiatrist and an outspoken critic of his peers, said the work of analysts and psychotherapists had more in common with that of magicians, semioticians, and sociologists.[2] Weekes explicitly agreed with Szasz and quoted approvingly of his 1961 book *The Myth of Mental Illness*, where he concluded that 'psychiatric interventions are aimed at moral, not medical problems'.[3]

To tell a patient, as Weekes did, that they could recover and then to tell them how to do it was just unthinkable for psychiatrists, according to Winston. Yet Hardy had been doing just this for years in Minnesota, building a reputation for successfully treating fearful patients.

When Hardy died in 1991, an obituary in *The New York Times* described him as a man who 'dissatisfied with the results of classical psychoanalysis ... broke with his Freudian training'.[4] There was no mention of Weekes among those who influenced him. Instead, two men were named — the well-known Dr Arnold Lazarus and Dr Joseph Wolpe.

According to Winston, Weekes' revelation that agoraphobia was a 'complication of having panic attacks was the huge contribution that saved so many people from unhelpful treatment with either psychodynamic or traditional cognitive behavioural therapy'.

Having grasped the power of Weekes' books and the thinking behind them, Winston went on to found what she calls the 'highly controversial Agoraphobia Clinic' in the outpatient department of the Sheppard and Enoch Pratt Hospital.

'The hospital community was sceptical, as psychoanalytic theory predicted that behavioural therapies would produce symptom substitution and the emergence of "deeper" conflict. This approach was considered simultaneously superficial and dangerous,' she recalls.

In later years, the clinic was vindicated and eventually became the Anxiety and Stress Disorders Institute of Maryland, as the early controversies died away. Weekes' six-word therapy, 'face, accept, float, and let time pass', was, along with her concept of first and second fear, 'just revolutionary', says Winston, who points out that Weekes anticipated by decades acceptance and commitment therapy (ACT) developed by the American clinical psychologist Steven Hayes.

Weekes' insights into the brain also proved prescient. Winston believes that Weekes understood the relationship between the mind and the body, the way the brain functions, and its fear circuitry well before anyone else. Her early insights are today supported by state-of-the-art brain tomography.

'In the last ten years, people have come to understand the fear circuitry in the brain in a way that they didn't before. What the neuroscientist Joseph LeDoux developed and disseminated everywhere was basically first fear/second fear. He hadn't heard of Claire Weekes either.'

Weekes had harnessed her wagon to the wider problem of what the contemporary textbooks may have called neurosis, although she would avoid such a judgemental term in favour of a medical description — nervous illness. Her descriptions were always suggestive of a temporal condition rather than a permanent state. She saw what could be called mental illness and mental health as a continuum.

The sexual revolution of the 1960s meant that the emotional freight of the repressed Victorian culture that had inspired Freud had been superseded. The very question of what was being treated was under assault. What was a mental disorder, and why was it 'mental'? Wasn't the brain involved as well? What exactly were the disorders, and how many were there? What was normal and what was not? Homosexuality, for example, was still defined as a disorder in the psychiatric manual, the *DSM*, until 1972.

In the 1970s, the law courts were taking less notice of psychiatric opinion, and often overruling expert psychiatric testimony recommending incarceration. Antiestablishment ideas were resurgent, and a counterculture extended into universities. The politics of the day did not suit psychiatry, and psychiatrists were accused of locking up people whose only problem was to not fit in.

The war in Vietnam further divided American psychiatrists, some of whom had worked for the military and who had asserted that, compared to WWII and the Korean War, where war neurosis had been left to fester, the military had anticipated the problem and created a treatment protocol that reduced evacuations for psychiatric reasons to less than 5 per cent of the total.[5] It was the fierce activism of the Vietnam Veterans Against the War that publicised the delayed massive trauma that afflicted so many returned soldiers.

A battle for the 'science' raged throughout this decade, and the arena was the *DSM-III*, control of which fell to the labellers — the splitters — led by Robert Spitzer, himself a psychiatrist, from Columbia University, in New York. Yet Spitzer challenged psychoanalysis and its putatively unscientific methods as he and his researchers took the lead in the revision of the professional manual.

He pushed for distinct diagnoses. For Spitzer, mental illnesses needed to be identified and named so that doctors could treat them. Cynics pointed out that pharmaceutical companies could design drugs to target such officially designated 'disorders', and the Boston conference that finalised the different categories for *DSM-III* was financed by Upjohn, the manufacturer of Xanax.

While he led the team that multiplied the number of mental disorders, Spitzer later expressed misgivings about the labelling trend he had championed, conceding the possibility that those critics who suggested *DSM-III* pathologised normal behaviour — for example, shyness — might be right. Ironically, it had been Spitzer who had originally helped to remove homosexuality from *DSM-II*.

Yet along with agoraphobia and panic disorder came a major new diagnostic category that was arguably more helpful, as it at least augured a formal recognition of the consequences of war service for individuals. The years of pressure from the Vietnam Veterans Against the War had led to the inclusion of a condition called post-traumatic stress disorder. Here, at last, was vindication for Grafton Elliot Smith and the many doctors who had urged governments to understand shell shock in WWI.

The profession still struggled with the idea that anxiety could lead to depression, a point made simply by Weekes, who preferred the term depletion, with the implied possibility of repletion. In her first book, *Self Help for Your Nerves*, she said depression was 'born from emotional fatigue'.[6] She described the feeling of the 'horse's hoof' on the chest but took a medical or biological view of what she saw: an exhausted nervous system. 'If you ... can view the body as temporarily depleted, rather than depressed, and understand that in time it can heal itself by recharging its emotional battery, hope comes into the picture.' It would be years before the profession caught up with the idea that anxiety and depression were linked, or, in the professional parlance, were comorbidities.

In 2012, Dr Thomas L. Schwartz attempted to introduce a program for 'treatment-resistant depression'. His goal was to focus on purely depressed patients who were not suffering from other comorbidities, but it became readily apparent that finding patients with 'only' major depressive disorder and without any other psychiatric comorbidities was almost impossible. Almost all had both depression and anxiety.

Fifty years after Weekes saw the linkage between the two, Schwartz wrote 'there have been very few studies on comorbid depression and anxiety and no FDA approval for a single medication treating these co-occurring, simultaneous disorders despite there being at least a 50% overlap in them in the general psychiatric population'.[7]

Weekes made the case for an environmental rather than genetic cause for depression:

> The mood of one member of the family can be too easily flattened by the depressed attitude of another member. Also, if several members of the family suffer with depression, other members can too easily become afraid that they too will eventually suffer from it. A sure way to become depressed is to be constantly frightened; fear exhausts and depression is so often an expression of emotional exhaustion.[8]

Weekes understood genetics, and if she wished to look for evidence, she could find it in her own family, but she resisted the determinism of a genetic explanation. Instead, she ended up on the side of the psychologists who favoured cognitive behaviour therapy as the first line of treatment, and against the proponents of the chemical-imbalance theory.

Yet there would be no tidy category into which she would fit or would ever be fitted. Like the scholars of old, she had a multidisciplinary approach to anxiety, and her own personal experience as a compass. Weekes' books addressed all of what the *DSM* had decided were a series of different disorders. Her treatment of all of them came back to the same 'simple but not easy' idea of acceptance rather than fighting.

Chapter 28

OLD AGE

Sometime in the early 1980s, an Australian psychiatrist paid a visit to Weekes at her Cremorne home. Gavin Andrews' intention was to pay homage, and it had taken him some time to get to this point.

Initially resistant to her writings, Andrews had found Weekes' self-help books 'terrible' and very 'patient oriented'. They didn't appeal to his scholarly inclinations; where was the scientific validation and evaluation? Why had she not completed a randomised controlled study? Frankly sceptical, he concluded that the advice was no more illustrious than that of a 'good grandmother'.

Andrews had a deep professional and scholarly interest in Weekes' subject, and, as a professor of psychiatry, had an international pedigree in the field. He had trained overseas in the 1950s, when the great promise of drugs to cure mental illness beckoned. Later, influenced by Dr Isaac Marks and his psychological work on anxiety in England, Andrews returned to Australia looking for a niche. Although psychiatrically trained, he eschewed drugs and psychoanalysis, and instead opted to practise CBT à la Marks, establishing the first anxiety clinic in his home country.

Over the years, he saw, with some envy, how Weekes' books were prominently displayed in airport newsstands around the world. He also noted some of his own patients 'had been helped by her books'. Slowly, he came around.

He knew Weekes had been on a difficult path. 'The College of Physicians must have thought she had moved too far outside the mainstream in respect of agoraphobia — after all she thought there was no need for medication in many cases, that people could cure themselves after reading her book, and … the book was on sale everywhere, even at airports — it was all too much really.'

It was Weekes' scepticism about drug treatment that inspired him to seek her out. He shared her resistance to the theory of a chemical imbalance in the brain.

Arriving at her Cremorne home, Andrews introduced himself to 'a little old lady without any of the grand dame who seemed pleased that someone had done her an honour by coming to see her'. He found 'an intelligent sympathetic person' and recalls he was on his best behaviour. It was a sort of 'ceremonial dance, and I knew that I was doing her an honour by going to see her because older people tend to get forgotten'. So why did he go? 'You can't have the Queen of the May retire and not go to throw garlands at her feet,' is his reply.

Some professionals were by now catching up with the fact that Weekes was offering something profoundly new and useful. Marks himself acknowledged her work in one of his many scholarly books. He deployed one of her colourful images of agoraphobia — more a showcase of the Weekes-family humour — 'a solitary figure, chewing vigorously on a candy, holding a dog leash in one hand and pushing her shopping cart in the other. This was Aggie Phobie who only went out after dark'.[1]

In Bradford, England, she was invited to speak at the Lynfield Mount Hospital. Psychiatrists from a nearby centre were under instructions from their director to boycott the event, but they turned up anyway and informed her of the ban.

Other psychiatrists in the UK and the US told her they would not start treating a patient until he or she had read one of her books. Dr William Sanderson, who was working in the 1980s in Dr David Barlow's anxiety clinic in the US, says patients would come in and 'tell me about the book'. He was surprised how many people found it, and he came to understand this work had provided 'an enormous resource to patients'.

A new edition of *Hope and Help for Your Nerves* was published in 1981, and, on the front cover, Ann Landers was quoted: 'This remarkable woman has helped many people. I recommend *Hope and Help for Your Nerves* with my whole heart.'

At White Plains in New York in the early 1980s, Weekes was a VIP guest and appreciated the respect and attention from professionals at the clinic. Typically, there was an offer of hospitality. Jean Easterbrook had been a patient of Dr Zane's, and on hearing that Dr Claire Weekes was visiting White Plains had decided, without consulting anyone, to ring her in Australia to invite her to stay in the home she shared with her mother. This was almost the perfect arrangement from Weekes' point of view. There was a photo taken of a very relaxed Weekes in the bedroom in which she stayed at Easterbrook's.

His exposure to White Plains and Weekes had already inspired Bob DuPont to change the direction of his career. Given Weekes' unique therapeutic offering and her pulling power, DuPont was keen to harness her talent to his fledgling Phobia Society of America, and he invited her to Washington in 1983 to host a special lecture at his Second Annual Meeting. 'She drew people from all over the United States,' DuPont recalled.

Curious about her own experience of anxiety, DuPont discovered to his surprise that she admitted to occasional attacks of panic at night. He expressed his sympathy, only to find her utterly uninterested in his well-intentioned words.

'My boy, you may be good with drug problems, but you have no talent for the treatment of anxiety,' she replied. 'What you call a panic attack is nothing but a few chemicals temporarily out of place in my brain. It means nothing to me, so your sympathy shows you don't understand the problem or the solution. Thus, I do not want or need your sympathy. It does not bother me. It is unimportant.'

This was the other side of Weekes — autocratic and undiplomatic. Yet this was the same woman who never failed to take phone calls from people in distress, who gave them her unstinting personal and professional support, and who told her niece Tita that 'it is only the really nice ones who get sick'.

Her patients and readers responded in kind. DuPont remembered that, the same year, 'an evening with Dr Claire Weekes' was held at White Plains in the clinic's treatment centre, and he had never seen any comparable therapeutic triumph. 'To walk with her through a group of people suffering from agoraphobia, virtually all of whom had really benefited from her books, was an experience like no other in my life,' DuPont said. 'People of all ages came up to her, many with tears in their eyes, pulled out their dogeared copies of one or the other of her books, and said something like: "thank you for making my life bearable. I never thought I would have the opportunity of seeing you myself and thanking you for what your work has meant to me and my family."'[2]

DuPont now put a proposition to Weekes. He would host an event where she could talk to some patients, and he would videotape the conversations. This would then be a powerful promotion for both her ideas and for his Phobia Society, which was helping educate the growing market for anxiety treatments.

Weekes agreed and DuPont set up the interviews. The videotape was made, and Weekes returned to Australia. Once at home, however, she had a complete change of heart, and immediately contacted DuPont. She had made a terrible mistake, she told him, and she wanted to stop the videotape being used in any form.

DuPont was shocked and distressed, pointing out that the Phobia Society had paid $10,000 to have it produced. He tried to talk her around, but Weekes was unmoved. The tape must be destroyed, and she would personally repay the $10,000. DuPont, greatly frustrated, was forced to accept her terms. Weekes had rejected a collaboration with someone who finally had genuine standing and experience to help her extend the market for her work.

The debacle was partly a by-product of her prior experience with business partners. Her experience with her agents in America, Yianitsas and Reich, had been so painful that she was wary of another joint venture. On top of that, and possibly more germane, was her anxiety about inviting further conflict, particularly with Reich, who claimed ownership of all the non-book copyright in the US through Worth Productions.

There was no Coleman to consult, and the stress of conflict had left its mark. That Weekes was now agitated was demonstrated by her willingness to pay $10,000 to DuPont to destroy the recording. Although she lived in a big house and had written bestselling books, she hadn't held a full-time job for nearly two decades, and, while comfortably well-off, was not a wealthy woman.

DuPont deeply regretted the destruction of the tape. He concluded that while Weekes had a brilliant gift, she could be a very difficult individual. Their personal relationship fractured, although DuPont continued to promote her work and recommend it to his patients.

Weekes' personal life was increasingly stressful. Dulcie had been diagnosed with dementia in 1979. She was now completely dependent. In her books, Weekes was always careful to distinguish between the simple anxiety state and one complicated by a very real 'problem', which she said might require the aid of a good counsellor. Now she was managing a set of ever more difficult problems, alone.

Weekes was almost as old as the century and without insulation. She was reluctant to face the implications of Dulcie's dementia, creating tension with those in the family who looked to her for support. As Dulcie deteriorated, an ageing Weekes was facing a burden that would become near intolerable.

Dementia offered infinite variations, and Dulcie had her own. She could go through 200 teabags, three litres of milk, and one kettle a week. Her daughter Tita, still living downstairs with her sons, was despairing and increasingly resentful that her aunt had spent so much time abroad, leaving her to manage her unmanageable mother. When at home, Weekes felt the pressure intensely. She had not anticipated dementia when she persuaded Dulcie to live upstairs.

Once, the strain felt so overwhelming that Weekes bolted, turning up on Lili's doorstep in the next suburb, repeating over and over, 'I just have to get away from Dulcie.' Lili and her husband, Nigel, made their own bed available to their ageing aunt, although she soon moved to another room. She stayed with them for ten days.

For total respite, there was always London. Skene Keating's Kensington apartment was her second home, and Weekes regularly escaped there.

In April 1982, Zane had written inviting her to give the guest lecture at the National Phobia Conference at White Plains. He was planning well ahead as it was scheduled for May 1983. Weekes was pleased with the invitation but was feeling her age and some uncomfortable emotions. She wrote back to Zane saying she was 'honoured and touched' but that much depended on her health. 'I'm now in my 80th year and sometimes still well enough to tackle anything, including a 40-hour plane journey to and from New York. However other times I'm too tired to go to the local store.'

She used a word, 'bewilderment', that any reader of her books would recognise. 'Old age,' she wrote to Zane, 'is certainly a bewilderment. It is a tantalising time to be alive because by 80 so many delightful hens have come home to roost, but one feels sometimes unable to go and collect the eggs!'

Weekes promised to come if she possibly could but urged him to have a fallback to ensure no 'embarrassing hiatus — no Dr Weekes'. She wanted an understudy. Again, she mentioned age. 'Never grow old. I'd be delighted to tell you how it all happened. In the meantime, I am trying to write my next book.'

She threw in a list of complaints: 'The mail is a heavy cross and the telephone (especially from USA) insistent. I also do all the shopping, and at the moment the cooking, and look after a sick sister.' To balance the querulous tone, she signed off on a positive note: 'all this is better than sitting knitting'.

The 1980s would not get any easier, even with those happy chickens coming home to roost. Her local publisher, Richard Walsh, the chief executive of A&R, had a high opinion of Weekes' work and wanted another book. The respectable, conservative Weekes and the highly creative Walsh had a steady, mutually rewarding collaboration. He felt the generational difference and suspects she may have disapproved of the fact that he had a medical degree but didn't practice. 'She may have thought that was unbelievable,' Walsh says. Yet they got on well. 'I found her very easy to deal with. She was very factual and very reliable.'

Walsh inherited Weekes as one of his authors, but, despite his history as a disruptor, there would be no changing her work or turning her upside down. A&R 'needed reprogramming', as he puts it, but Walsh appreciated both the quality of her work and her market appeal. Why change the formula? They had a formal relationship, given their age difference, and Walsh viewed Weekes 'very much as the lady doctor'. Better still, she gave him little trouble, having no need for any duchessing, unlike some of his other authors.

Walsh was not a publisher who felt he had to approve of every book he published, and he admitted commissioning plenty that he regarded with misgivings, even when they sold well. Weekes' books were in a different category, and she genuinely earned the audience she achieved, in his opinion. Like so many others she would come across in her work, there was a personal edge to Walsh's professional regard. He had recommended her books to several of his friends, and, to his 'great gratification', they were extremely well received. Weekes' books had been '*really* useful', he was told.

Just as relevant was that Walsh found the books helpful himself. Until the age of 45, he had suffered from migraines. He believed that one source of his creative powers was his manic bursts of energy, but they were regularly followed by blinding headaches. 'My form of depression,' was how he described them.

They were savage. 'I felt absolutely like a tortoise on its back, because I was used to being a man of action, but suddenly I was absolutely hopeless. There was nothing I could do. I wasn't the sort of person who would try meditation, but, instead of lying there and thinking, "this is frightful, why doesn't it go away," I rolled with absolutely accepting it.' Acceptance worked.

When you are on a good thing, stick to it. Walsh knew her audience wanted *more*, and he proposed the new book be titled *More Help for Your Nerves*. Weekes was paid an advance of $16,000, a significant publishing commitment in 1983. But how much 'more' was there to say on the topic, particularly given Weekes' advanced age and diminished energy?

One answer was to limit the amount of fresh writing that had to be done, and so the book included several interviews, some articles Weekes had produced for self-help groups abroad, and a speech. This helped ease the load.

As usual, Weekes employed direct speech, writing in the first person. More emphasis was put on time — how long it took for nerves to recover and how setbacks were inevitable. 'Time must pass, always give it time.' And there was more on setbacks and the importance of an understanding that had been 'earned'.

> For as long as memory brings suffering, doubting complete recovery is natural. Recovery means being able to look full faced at memory, prepared to accept any suffering it may bring. Complete cure does not necessarily mean absence of symptoms, although it can. It means knowing how to cope with the symptoms stress may present, at any time, any place. Being able to cope is not only possible it is inevitable, when recovery has been earned by the sufferer's own effort based on understanding.

Weekes' original prescriptions remained unchanged, but the book extended the repertoire of suffering — the fear of setbacks, the morning's 'knife edge', the fed-up family, hypochondria, the fear of being alone, whether depression could be inherited. Writing over 20 years after her first book, she addressed ageing and death. Although she admitted to DuPont that she herself found old age 'bewildering', she made no such admissions in print. Instead, there was a chapter called 'More Bewilderments Cleared'.

Under the subhead 'Old age or nervous illness?', Weekes said:

> Your question has been asked of me many times. I have found that if the questioner stops trying to fathom how much fatigue is the result of nervous illness and how much of old age, and instead does what he can within the

limits of his present strength without thrashing himself too severely with doubt and bewilderment, he is surprised how much he can gradually do. Our bodies have great recuperative powers if we remove tension — even in our 80s. I have proved this on myself.[3]

As for death:

I could tell you that 'what can't be cured must be endured' and so it must, but how to endure a fear of death that may haunt for years — sometimes a lifetime — while yet being prepared to face death that actually comes? That is the point. Sudden death gives no time for its contemplation, so why should we fear it? While some people are concerned with sudden death, most are concerned with death that may come gradually, when they are old. Here again, I speak as a doctor, I have rarely attended a person actually dying that realised that he, or she, was dying.

A few do but very few. Nature blunts the edge of her sword; even during the years before our death nature helps us; our habits, our demands on life change. At 20, the weekend means activity — dinner and dance and tennis; at 70, we'd rather sit by the fire and read. Activity naturally slows down. If we are prepared to go along with nature as willingly as possible, she will make a death rather like a birth — we will be the star performer but we will be unaware of the performance. I don't say that there may not be suffering for many during those long months — even years — but here again, age dulls feeling to a certain extent; inevitability brings its own anaesthesia.[4]

Working on another book lifted her spirits, and Weekes decided she felt capable of delivering the main speech at the 1983 annual National Phobia Conference, sponsored by both Zane's clinic and DuPont's Phobia Society. In March, she wrote to Zane to let him know she would be there.

> Thank you for the program. So far, I'm coming. Be booking my seat next week. Of course, the $500 will be very welcome as the fares have grown wings and there is no catching them. I thank you for your thought.
>
> I have a good housekeeper at last who will be able to hold the fort while I'm away. My book is almost finished — I finished the second draft and need only to correct it and have the final draft typed which I'll be bringing with me. I go into much more detail about the complications of certain aspects of nervous illness. When it has been published, which will be, I hope, at the end of the year, I will return to America to go on television. In the meantime I will stay in London.

England was offering the prospect of significant, serious publicity. The BBC had invited her to give a series of ten-minute interviews to run over several weeks. It was scheduled for September later that same year. These were some of the delightful chickens that had come home to roost.

On 7 May 1983, Weekes delivered her address at the Fourth National Phobia Conference, at White Plains Hospital. Her speech was titled 'Treatment of Phobias: the role of the professional and the paraprofessional'. She wanted her audience to understand one key ingredient for recovery and why 'a treatment based mainly on belief is in danger of working only temporarily'. She had been refining the idea of the inner voice — a key departure between her work and that of professionals she criticised for their top-down approach.

> For recovery the sufferer must have, deep within himself, a special voice that says during any setback or dark moment, 'it's all right; you've been here before, you know the way out. You can do it again. It works, and you know it works!' That voice speaks with authority and brings comfort only when it has been earned by the sufferer himself and it can be earned only by making the symptoms and experiences that torture no longer matter. No longer mattering is the key. It is not a question of some method of treatment, spiriting misery away, anaesthetising it. It is a question of the symptoms, the experiences, no longer mattering.[5]

New York psychologist Bob Ackerman was in attendance that day, and he remembers that, at the very end of her speech, she asked for the tape recorder, always turned on for her speeches, to be turned off. She then told this audience of professionals about her personal experience, all those years ago as a young woman studying for her doctorate.

A few days later, she discovered that a presentation she had agreed to give to a group of Zane's nervously ill patients would be a much larger affair than she had anticipated. Zane had advertised the event, and Weekes found herself in front of another full house. He introduced her as a 'real pioneer' in the field but explained to the audience how indifferent the profession was to her achievements, harking back to her speech in New York in 1977 when he was struck by 'the depth of her observations and the lack of appreciation, it seemed to me, by most of the audience of what she had to say'.

Her books were a revelation. As a psychiatrist, psychoanalytically trained, 'I knew this was something different: she was coming to us from where the patient is, and not from on top, where we were telling the patient what it's all about — why you are the way you are. But she was listening to what people say.' Zane added that, over the years, he had consistently heard people tell him that they 'never believed there was anybody who could understand me that way'.

Weekes had prepared no speech, anticipating a question-and-answer session with a small group of people, so she was at a bit of a loss. She solved her problem by conversing with an imaginary patient sitting in a chair next to her, overwhelmed by not being able to cope with the simplest responsibilities. 'She wasn't going mental,' Weekes said of this patient, 'she wasn't even strange — she was just an ordinary person whose physical demands to cope with stress weren't being met.'

Then, for two hours, Weekes answered questions. She spoke on the chemical-imbalance theory of the brain. She was a believer, but only in her own chemical-imbalance theory. 'In my opinion, nervous illness comes first, and chemical imbalance follows. Fix the nervous illness and the chemical imbalance will right itself.' However, she explicitly drew a line between the anxiety state and 'illnesses that have a known chemical imbalance, such as manic depression and postnatal depression'.

Towards the end of the presentation, her professional guard dropped. 'Now I must tell you that you can panic even though you have no fear of it. That's almost like a confession, isn't it.'

A question about guilt triggered a rush of personal reminiscences. 'How do I deal with feelings of guilt? Oh, boy! Well, sometimes you don't, and I tell you when you age you look back, and I said to myself to cheer myself up one day, "now I'm going to try to think of some of the good things that I have done," and you know, I couldn't, I just couldn't! I tried to write them down and look at them. But you know you think of all the things you should not have done!'

What was it that so consumed her with guilt? There was a clue in some later words she offered on the same subject.

> If it involves other people it's difficult isn't it? And I'll tell you one thing: if you have an old mother or an old father, or a relative who is sick, be as nice and kind to them as you can, because when they're dead you can't bring them back to tell them how much you love them, or how you wish you had been kind to them. It's terribly important to show old people that you love them *now*.[6]

Of whom was she thinking? Fan, Ralph, or Beth?

Chapter 29

THE BBC AND A BLIZZARD
OF LETTERS

Marcel Aurousseau died on 22 August 1983. At the age of 92, this was not unexpected but had special poignancy for Weekes. Everyone in her family knew, or knew of, Marcel, the 'perfect man' she nearly married, and they all knew her oldest friend, Cecily.

After Coleman had died, the Aurousseaus' Balgowlah home had provided Weekes with a refuge, and an intellectual haven in an otherwise barren landscape. Their three lives had remained entwined. A clue to the depth of her attachment to these two individuals was the dedication in Weekes' final book, in the year before she died. 'To Marcel and Cecily Aurousseau. There is a lifetime of meaning in those two names.'

Another family tragedy followed. Her eldest niece, Frances, lost one of her three daughters in a road accident. It was a terrible time for Frances, who had also suffered through a divorce, and she remembers her aunt counselling against her frenzied activity as she battled the insanity of grief.

Meanwhile, Dulcie pottered along, becoming more and more baffled. This was stressful enough, but Weekes found her escape route was slowly closing over. When she headed to London, she ran into the same problem she was fleeing in Sydney. Joyce Skene Keating was showing signs of dementia, too, and, as her children became increasingly concerned about her welfare, they also looked to Weekes for support and advice. Her unassailable position as doctor and matriarch, which had assured her primacy, now came with expectations that she found difficult to handle.

She had tried to run, and now she tried to hide. Just as she had denied the reality of Dulcie's mental disarray, she found it difficult to accept the deterioration in the health of her London friend, so obviously struggling with her dual responsibilities as a magistrate and as a distribution agent for the audiotapes in Weekes' non-book business.

Yet as the unsteady props under her personal life wobbled, Weekes' fame continued to spread, which only increased the pressure on her international business. The BBC interviews represented another significant opportunity. The six planned television interviews were being researched and produced by Fran Groves, who was working for the BBC's new flagship daytime television program, *Pebble Mill at One*.

Groves had tripped across the work of Weekes by chance and, like so many others, found it had a particularly personal meaning. 'I was working in a very high-pressured daytime program, where we went live for 45 minutes every day. I was under pressure generally and was having panic attacks and was not able to cope with them really,' she says.

Groves was specialising in health coverage, and her proposal for a series of talks, to be broadcast weekly, was accepted as a segment for *Pebble Mill at One*. When she finally contacted Weekes, Groves was captivated by her sense of humour and deep compassion, describing her as 'a colossus of calm'.

When Weekes agreed to the interviews, she was asked to

nominate someone who could tell the story of how she had cured them of serious nervous illness. As the segment producer, Groves wanted to demonstrate the power of Weekes' work. About half a dozen people were approached — one with phobias, one with obsessions, one with depression, one with agoraphobia. But this was the 1980s, when mental health was, if not taboo, then some-what shaming. Nobody wanted this sort of exposure. Finally, Weekes called in a favour and asked Anne Turner from Yorkshire, who was not delighted with the prospect, but agreed to sign on. Turner remained indebted to Weekes for her life-saving inter-vention in the early 1970s, when she was facing the unacceptable prospect of a lobotomy.

'Everybody chickened out except me, so I was the patient,' says Turner. 'And I didn't even want to go public on it like that. You didn't talk about these things at that time. It was a very big thing.'

The interviews were a very big thing for Weekes, too. Her usually unbreakable confidence was brittle. 'At 81, one is very open to doubt!' She wasn't afraid of forgetting what happened over the last 40 years but feared forgetting what she had said 'half a minute ago'.

The programs were live, which Weekes found particularly daunting, and so she took the precaution of practising in detail for six weeks before the first broadcast, walking the streets of London, reciting each talk over and over again. 'This preparation did not fail,' she declared later.

The BBC had its features department in Birmingham, and Weekes travelled there accompanied by Skene Keating, whom Groves remembers as 'a true sort of lady' but also a 'bag of nerves'. Groves was convinced that Skene Keating would do anything Weekes asked of her. Skene Keating's son, Paul, allows that although his mother was troubled, Weekes had improved her symptoms.

And Skene Keating was not without her own authority. Groves asked Weekes if she had ever had any trauma herself, and Weekes had just started to answer when Joyce jumped in: 'Claire! No!'

Paul Skene Keating believes his mother was very protective of her great friend, yet Groves saw a woman in distress over her responsibility for Weekes. When Weekes misplaced her handbag only a few minutes before she was due to go on air and turned to her for help, Groves noticed how badly this rattled Skene Keating, and remarked later, 'She just couldn't cope with that much stress.'

The interviews were broadcast in late 1983. Weekes was in confessional mode. Finally, she admitted what anyone who read her books discerned, that her medical expertise was anchored by personal experience. She told her own story of nervous illness, the misdiagnosed tuberculosis, the uncaring doctor who refused assistance when her heart was racing, the doctorate produced in a state of constant, overwhelming anxiety, the respite on the boat to London, and the recurrence of all the terrible symptoms once on land. She spoke of her friend's advice, but Marcel was once again camouflaged as John. She explained that, when she later became a medical practitioner and went into general practice, 'I became very sympathetic towards patients who came to me in an anxiety state because I knew what it was like to be in one.'

She was buoyantly talking of cure, but when presenter Marian Foster asked her, 'You're actually saying that people can be cured?' her answer was carefully nuanced.

'Of course, I have no fear of using the word "cured". I get a little sad when I hear some therapists saying that nervous illness cannot be cured, only relieved.' However, Weekes added that 'it can be cured as long as the person who has suffered is prepared to live with the memory of that suffering and knows how to deal with its recurrences. If memory brings the feelings back, the feelings of suffering, the sufferer may feel sure he's sick again and his therapist will often agree and tell him that he's not yet cured and obviously they haven't got to the real cause of it.'

Here she made an interesting parallel with losing a loved one, and surely she was thinking of Coleman. 'If you lose someone you love, you often suffer when you think of them. We can't say to our heart "don't suffer!" We have to live with the feelings in our heart, and, despite the aching, we do live on.'

So with nervous illness, the same applied. It was impossible to say you must never suffer again. 'We can't obliterate memory. Of course he will remember his suffering, but that does not mean he is not cured. That means only that memory is up to its old tricks.'

The audience response was immediate, overwhelming, and unprecedented. The avalanche of letters following the six-part series busted the postbox of the BBC, which was forced to employ outworkers and rent space to accommodate the mail. The BBC's business manager, Ann Fitch, wrote to Groves saying the broad-caster had been 'receiving 200–600 letters a day since the start of the series 5 weeks ago. It's therefore estimated that there has been a total of around 10–12,000 letters ... from all over Great Britain, men and women and some professional people: doctors and psychiatrists.' They had to pay for extra secretarial help to cope with the personal letters.

Inspired by this huge response, Groves and Foster decided to turn the interviews into a video that could be circulated widely and would provide a permanent record. The BBC allowed them to use their facilities, and further conversations between Foster and Weekes were recorded. Four hours of interviews were then edited down to just over an hour.

The BBC agreed to release the copyright to Weekes, who signed a contract to pay the public broadcaster 25 per cent of net income from sales. A company, Pacific Recordings, was established by Groves, Foster, and Weekes to market the video, and Weekes paid for the production of a master tape.

She told her new partners that she had a wealthy American supporter who was the financial backer for the project, and, at some stage, she managed to contact Reich to interest him in her latest venture. A year later, Weekes wrote to the Australian Tax Office informing them that the company that she ran with Steven Reich had 'incurred great expense by buying the rights to certain medical videotapes in the United States and England'. The American master tape had cost $16,000, and the English, £1800. This had been paid, she told the ATO, by Steven Reich from Florida.

Accepting the money from Reich was a mistake, for in doing so she completely lost control of the American end of the business. She was now in his debt, and he felt entitled to do what he wished with the video he had paid for.

There were tensions in England as well. When she could no longer ignore the fact that Skene Keating wasn't coping, Weekes turned to the loyal Anne Turner, imploring her to step in. The ailing Skene Keating was stripped of the job; at least that's how Paul Skene Keating sees it, feeling the matter was handled insensitively.

Turner herself had misgivings. She knew the price Skene Keating had paid, because she had heard it firsthand from her. Whenever Weekes was in London, Turner would visit, and she had spent a lot of time at Skene Keating's residence.

'Before she was poorly,' Turner recalls, 'Joyce had been trying to set up a business to handle Dr Weekes' work. And it had caused a great deal of stress with her family, as it does because it takes over everything. And she said, "If ever I can't do this, Anne, if she ever asks you, do be careful before you accept because it causes an awful lot of trouble." And I could see for her what trouble it caused, because Joyce put everything first for Dr Weekes. Her family came second and that caused trouble with them.'

Despite the warning, Turner agreed to take on the job. Weekes was prepared to pay for the service, but Turner was not particularly interested in the money. She regarded Weekes as a mother figure. Their relationship had deepened, particularly after Coleman died, and they spent many hours on the phone between Australia and England.

By the time the video was finally ready, Turner was effectively Weekes' business manager in Britain and handling all the audio work that had been Skene Keating's responsibility. She came under pressure from Weekes to get involved in promoting the video — and felt squeezed by Weekes on the one hand, and her husband on the other. Bob Turner wanted his wife to pull back. He had not been well and would die of cancer a few years later. Yet Turner viewed the other two women, Groves and Foster, as usurpers, and believed she should be in charge. Her husband eventually complained to Weekes, whose response was to press Groves and Foster to involve Turner, a proposal they resisted.

Once again, Weekes had somehow conjured up a vexing business mess. In the end, the two BBC broadcasters pulled out of the whole endeavour, leaving the responsibility for selling and distributing the video to Turner.

At the same time as she authorised Turner to take over Pacific Recordings, Weekes gave a charity permission to make use of her audio cassettes. She had approached Amber Lloyd, who had set up Relaxation for Living in 1972, because the charity relied heavily on her work. Relaxation for Living would take over the distribution of the cassettes in the UK.

Though Weekes had insisted to the BBC that Reich would be 'an enthusiastic distributor of the videocassettes', it was a sign of the times that she just wanted a verbal contract with Relaxation for Living. 'Dr Weekes had so much trouble with Steve Reich from America, she refused to sign any more contracts,' says Turner.

What was left out of this was an understanding that Relaxation for Living were required to pay Weekes a percentage of all monies they received for selling the recordings.[1] Once Amber Lloyd retired, Relaxation for Living morphed into corporate stress management schemes but continued to market and distribute the cassettes. As a result of these unorthodox arrangements, Weekes ended up with a slew of informal agreements that would be left to be unpicked by her heirs.

Though she made no financial gain from the video debacle, presenter Marian Foster was a beneficiary in a different way. She never suffered from nervous illness, but the video took some time to make, and, when Weekes saw her after two years had elapsed, the doctor's eye was still in focus.

'In those final interviews, she noticed that I had changed since she last saw me, and diagnosed that I had developed an overactive thyroid condition,' says Foster. 'She organised specialist treatment for me. I asked her how she knew, and she said lots of people went "hyper" during the war years, and she had learned to spot the symptoms. So I have a great deal to thank her for, and feel privileged to have known such a wonderful person.'

The thyroid, as Weekes would know, was one of the ductless glands.

Chapter 30

THE SOUND OF CLOSING DOORS

The last ten years of Weekes' life were in her own words 'especially almost impossible'. The only relief from the pressures of life, health, family, and the growing list of unmanageable business partners was that people continued to buy her books. Many of those who discovered the first book in 1962 were, however, like the author, beginning to feel their age.

In a radio interview with Marian Foster in Britain soon after the television series, Weekes spoke of the value of occasionally tranquillising 'grandma', with whom she presumably identified. 'As we get older, it's almost as if our nervous system more easily gets sensitised. You must surely have met grandma, who, although she loves the boys, can stand them only for a short while when they come to visit her? She soon retreats into her bedroom. Now if grandma had a mild tranquiliser when the boys arrived, she might even enjoy the visit.'

Weekes expressed the view that tranquillisers had 'their part to play, especially, as I have said, for old people. After all, as we get old, we may lose teeth — sometimes all of them — much of our hearing, and sight; we might also lose some of our ability to take things calmly.'

In 1984, *More Help for Your Nerves* was published. In the dedication, she rounded up all those she had been closest to in her life. Remarkably, in a list of those who were either family or whom she regarded as such, she included Steven Reich.

> To my sister, Dulcie Maclaren, for her courage and love; to my friends, Joyce Skene Keating, JP, Irene Appleton and Steven Reich, for their great effort and devotion to the work and to the memory of Elizabeth Coleman, who always put obligation before inclination and love and loyalty before all else.

Her US publishers had paid her an advance of $250,000 for the book, a very big number at the time.[1] Almost 30 years later, and 20 years after she died, her heirs were still receiving significant royalty payments as her books steadily sold. In 2017, Apple iBooks counted her at number 12 in their top-selling books in her category, health and wellbeing. She came in three spots after Dale Carnegie's *How to Win Friends and Influence People*, another self-help survivor.

A newly published book meant more travel, more promotional tours, which was now becoming problematic. When Weekes was away, Tita became more and more agitated about bearing the burden of her mother's care. She had two teenage boys on her hands as well as her own difficulties to contend with.

Dulcie may have been in her final decline, but she did not lose her playfulness. Tita's sons would come home from work and find themselves drenched by a bucket of water thrown from the top floor by their grandmother, who had been waiting for them to return. Dulcie's grandsons were amused, but, when Weekes was abroad in 1985, Dulcie's daughters decided to put their mother into a nursing home. Weekes paid the bill.

The family often made assumptions about her finances, given her success and her willingness to pay for her extended family when necessary. On one occasion, Tita's sons, Adam and Jason, looked to her for money. As schoolboys, they demonstrated an early flair for entrepreneurial effort, if not success, and organised a dance party at one of Sydney's largest venues, the Hordern Pavilion. Adam had saved $5000, and their aunt lent them another $5000. The money was lost, and Adam remembers this with regret. Tita says she demanded her sons repay their aunt, but Weekes 'never would take it'. It took some years, until he worked in the creative industries himself, but Adam later understood what had been asked of a woman who may not have been as rich as they all thought.

The pattern of generosity that began in the 1950s continued over the years, and, as Weekes' fame still grew, and her book sales with it, so did other's expectations. In her last decade, she found this occasionally distressing. She had no children herself but a small platoon of would-be dependents. She didn't always understand how to slice the pie, or how to refuse to serve it. The quality of restraint so effective in her professional life proved less so in the face of others with less self-control. The queen of the castle was now an ageing monarch.

When she returned to Australia in 1985, Weekes at least had Dulcie off her hands. This meant the upstairs apartment was empty, but Tita was still living downstairs and was always at home. Weekes had some domestic help and had engaged the mother of one of Tita's friends to prepare lunch for her daily, and she later employed Pat Ryder from Dial an Angel to provide companionship and secretarial duties. Yet the old robust Weekes was not entirely missing in action — she was planning another overseas trip.

At the age of 80, she had worried about the long flight to New York; at 83, she accepted another invitation from Zane to be the guest speaker at White Plains Hospital Phobia Clinic in New York in March 1986. Called 'An Evening with Dr Weekes', she was billed by the clinic as one of the great names in the treatment of phobias and a pioneer in the study of irrational fears and how to overcome them. Doreen Powell, who worked at White Plains Hospital, saw again her personal pulling power. 'We had a full house and people were standing in the aisles and corridors to express their gratitude for her help.'

In the same month, Weekes appointed Al Zuckerman from Writers House as her US literary agent, to handle her three contracts with Hawthorn, which had been taken over by E.P. Dutton, which itself licensed Bantam Books to publish them. Bantam now had her three earlier titles and were about to publish her fourth.

Correspondence between Zuckerman and Bantam incidentally revealed that Weekes' deal with Reich had gone off the rails. One of the ways in which Weekes had publicised her private audio and video business had been to get her publishers to publicise them in the books. Bantam had ceased this cross-promotion against her wishes. She suspected that it was because Reich, who was obliged to pay the publishers 5 per cent of his receipts, may not have done so.

Weekes was in the awkward position of asking Zuckerman to tell Bantam that she 'did not know this for a fact' and 'she would welcome any information on this which you could supply'. She had lost control of Reich and Worth Productions. She couldn't even reach him and now had only second-hand information, which included, bafflingly, that Reich had commenced medical studies in Washington.

The confusion over rights was particularly frustrating as Ann Landers had promised to promote the cassettes if only she could get hold of them. Weekes knew enough about Reich's temper and his belief that he had total ownership of the US copyright to get them to Landers in any other way.

She continued to struggle with Reich. He remained elusive. She received no payments from him and over her last decade met a steady stream of complaints from people who had tried, but failed, to purchase any of her audio recordings.

In a letter to Doreen Powell, she complained vigorously about her problems with him. The White Plains clinic was keen to get hold of all her audio and video products, but the only contact point anyone, including Weekes, had for Reich was a post-office box.

'They are still working, although heaven knows what is happening to Steven Reich who was supposed to run it for me,' she wrote to Powell. 'When I wanted to get somebody else to do this he threatened to take me to court. He has been ill again and I suspect still is. I'll send him a copy of your letter to stir him up. I can't reach him by phone although I have been trying almost daily.'

Weekes was completely defeated, but spared Doreen the details, concluding with: 'So I'm afraid you will have only that address to give. If you have any more complaints could you send them all to me? Then I should really attack him. It is a long story.'

In 1986, she was invited to appear on *The Late Late Show*, hosted by Gay Byrne in Dublin, Ireland. In a letter to her family, written in July, she boasted that 'within one week [of this interview] my books were on the bestseller list'. As for her non-book resources, at least Weekes had the loyal, reliable Anne Turner handling these in the United Kingdom.

From London, she wrote tenderly to Tita back in Sydney touching lightly on some of the pressures in the family: 'your letter made me happy — to think you are getting to know Esther and Brian better. I'm especially glad that he is beginning to appreciate you.'

With Dulcie in the nursing home, Brian and Esther would

regularly stay in Weekes' home, whether she was there or not, and so had more contact with Tita. Weekes was increasingly sentimental about these family ties. Family counted, and Tita mattered particularly. Weekes wanted her brother — who bullied his wife and children and was so often savagely critical of those around him — to see what she saw in her favourite niece.

She told Tita she had 'managed to get a Pinter for you' (a copy of one of Harold Pinter's plays that was out of print in Australia) as well as buying her 'a lovely pepper grinder — polished wood with a silver base — beautiful'. Weekes was still busily planning the future, and one that included Tita.

> When I come home, I will try to persuade you to have
> a trip over here — via USA — but to fit in with your
> work — a vacation I mean. I think of Dulcie daily and
> long to see her. She is still very lovable, and I miss her,
> My love, darling.

Weekes was overly optimistic about future travel. This would be her last trip. The impossible years were winding up. Another door was slamming shut. Skene Keating could no longer offer a refuge from any trouble in Sydney. Weekes had spent 25 years coming and going from the Skene Keating home, staying for months, and sometimes for half the year. Then she just stopped. Her age and circumstances meant she no longer had the strength herself to cope with her friend's condition.

Back in Sydney, Weekes' own health became more of an issue. Her redoubtable energy levels were flagging, her digestive problems troubled her, and she was taking tablets for blood pressure.

Here, there were more reminders of mortality. Brian had not been well for some time, but though he and Esther now lived in the Blue Mountains — over an hour's driving time from Sydney

— they still managed to get down to stay with her from time to time. Weekes was grateful for the company, yet Brian saw his elder sister's vulnerability, and his own, which he captured in his pungent prose in a letter to his daughter Barbara.

> We were going to Auntie Claire's, to empty chairs, spilt baby powder and wrecked Venetians [blinds] on the front veranda but with a beautiful view of the city across the harbour. Ease up Dad! You can't handle all this bottom-of-the-guts self-pity.[2]

Chapter 31

A BLOW TO THE BRAIN

If the previous few years had been difficult, 1987 marked a brutal turning point. In the middle of the year, Weekes saw her doctor for nothing more complicated than the routine health check required by the New South Wales roads and transport authority to verify that, at the age of 84, she was capable of driving.

She had just stepped out of the surgery when she collapsed on the footpath. Fortuitously, it was directly opposite one of Sydney's biggest teaching hospitals, the Royal North Shore, and so there was no delay in treatment, which was urgently required as she had hit her head. The resulting subdural haematoma, or bleed on the brain, was often caused by head injuries, and threatened brain damage if not treated. Weekes required an operation.

For almost a week, she lay comatose in a hospital bed. Her niece Lili visited daily and, sitting beside her aunt, would ask her to squeeze her hand if she could hear her. Eventually, Lili got a little squeeze in response, and, when Weekes was finally capable of conversation, she asked the same question over and over: 'Do you love me, Lil, do you love me, do you love me?'

Lili found this strange. Weekes knew she was loved. However, Lili understood her aunt was not dazed by drugs or somehow mentally bereft, and guessed she was frightened. Weekes did not believe in God. He or she would not save her, but Weekes knew the power of love as she had had it all her life, in uncommon quantities. She wanted it now.

The timely hospitalisation meant Weekes escaped brain damage but only to enter the mysterious ageing zone called frailty. As a doctor, she knew the road ahead, and was now rattled as well as vulnerable. Her blood pressure had been a problem for years. No longer was she capable of the systematic work that had a special significance for her, given her emphasis on the importance of what she called 'occupation'. Not so long before, she had written to Doreen Powell at White Plains offering sympathy for some of her troubles, adding that 'work and time' were the main helpers. Weekes had little of either left.

Discharged from hospital, it was obvious that she needed more help at home. Instead, her life was to about to get shaken by family conflicts, troubles, dramas, and jealousies. Just when she needed peace, quiet, and care, she was confronting great turbulence. Ironically, another bout of bad news would deliver her a carer.

Earlier that year, Brian had been diagnosed with an acoustic neuroma, a benign tumour in the inner ear that threatened to press on the brain. By the time it was discovered, it was very big, and surgery carried the risk of facial palsy. Brian dithered and wrote to his daughter.

> I said to [your] Mum as I wandered by her bed with her bed covered in Woman's Days and other stuff, I said: 'I feel so lost, just so lost.' She looked up and said 'what have you lost?' I said 'I've lost my operation. Perhaps I should have had it.' She said, 'with all that facial paralysis?' I felt more tangled up.

Finally, Brian opted for the surgery in Sydney. He and Esther moved in with Weekes for the duration. He was on the operating table for 13 hours, nearly died, and had to be resuscitated. Afterwards, he struggled with walking and his fine motor skills disappeared completely, effectively ending his artistic endeavours — he had held his first major art exhibition two years prior. This did nothing for his mood.

Soon after Brian's operation, Weekes hit her head on the footpath. When she was discharged from hospital, it fell to Esther to look after them both. Weekes got the companionship and help in the home she needed and wanted, although Esther was alert to the risk that Weekes would become increasingly dependent on her.

Brian came as close as Weekes got to intellectual companionship. Esther was content to stay in the background, working, as Coleman had done for years. Their presence was not an unmixed blessing. Brian still sharpened his bad temper on his wife, and his crass humour had to be tolerated, but that was nothing compared to the moods.

Yet Weekes loved Esther particularly, and, as they aged, they spent more time together. After the brother and sister recuperated, they moved between each other's houses with Weekes occasionally staying with them in the Blue Mountains, and Brian and Esther with her in Sydney.

Inevitably, the burden was too heavy for Esther, who struggled to manage the household and support two ageing individuals in poor health. She and Brian moved into a retirement village on the Northern Beaches. Brian was admitted into the nursing home while Esther lived in assisted accommodation in the same facility.

Weekes was horrified at the thought of institutional life and insisted on remaining in her home. But who would look after her? She had no children, but she did have money. As it turned out, Brian's eldest daughter, Penny, now in her 40s, was struggling financially. Her doctor husband had been jailed for fraud and they had lost the family home. It had been a large harbourside mansion not far from Weekes, but, in the way of forced sales, it incurred no profit as the market happened to be flat. Sydney property was famous for making investors rich, but individuals could find themselves occasionally on the wrong side of the cycle.

It was an irony that Penny, as a lifelong Labor supporter, found herself a victim of the economic downturn that Labor treasurer Paul Keating would later infamously describe as the 'recession that Australia had to have'. Although she had dramatically downsized from her huge family home to a small inner-city cottage, interest rates rose to 17 per cent in the late 1980s. Penny, unable to handle the repayments, lost the cottage, too, and was thrown back into the rental market.

According to Penny, it was Esther, fearing the burden of inheriting an ailing Weekes, who suggested that she move in with her aunt, who needed both help and companionship. Everyone knew Weekes was nervous at night and liked the security of someone with her. Conversation and company were vital. Penny needed accommodation and so the proposal was put to Weekes, who agreed to the arrangement.

In November 1988, Penny moved into 37 Milson Road, Cremorne. The arrangement turned out to be far from perfect. Two adult women who had lived apart most of their lives, one frail and dependent, the other under pressure, was not optimal. Tita wasn't happy with the new arrangements either.

The relationship between Penny and her aunt had never been particularly close. In some ways, this was surprising, as they had the most in common. Penny had started a medical degree, married a doctor who himself came from a medical family, and eventually graduated with honours as a clinical psychologist, specialising in anxiety and depression. Yet their overlapping interests offered no bridge to a closer relationship.

There were stressful dramas to endure as upstairs and downstairs juggled various family pressures. Not long after, Tita moved out and went to live in a nearby boarding house, leaving her boys behind. Weekes was devastated when Tita cut all contact.

Weekes was left in the care of Penny and the paid daytime help, but Penny was working full-time and had her own concerns beyond Cremorne. With Tita out of reach, Weekes spent far more time alone, and in fragile health. Lili was in full-time employment, and Cecily Aurousseau was homebound.

Although Weekes may have occasionally mismanaged the pressures around her, there were some that were, in her own words, 'simply impossible'. She was no longer in charge, and nothing worked exactly as she wished. She told Pat Ryder that she had lost control. 'I have always been a person who has been in command … and now I feel like an old woman.'

Tita says, 'She had been at the helm, she had steered the ship, she had driven the crew, and then the rudder broke.'

Chapter 32

EYES ON THE PRIZE

By 1988, Weekes felt besieged. Weakened by her fall and the subsequent surgery, she described the next 18 months as 'a stormy postoperative period — not pleasant at all'.[1] In the years after Coleman died, she would regularly wake at 4.00 a.m., bang on the floorboards to alert Tita, who also struggled with insomnia, and who would then come upstairs. They would talk until dawn. Even that comfort was now gone.

Weekes' remaining consolation was her friends abroad, and she rang them regularly to confide in them. They became her lifeline, and she relied on this extensively, venting her woes and any frustrations to Anne Turner in England and another patient-turned-believer, Charlotte Rudeau, in America, who, despite her geographical distance, now took a central place in Weekes' life.

Rudeau, who lived in Florida, credited Weekes with curing her of panic attacks in the late 1960s, when she had been in her early 30s. At the time, Charlotte was married to a writer, theatrical entrepreneur, and restaurant manager with whom she had two children. After a late night organising a big-name act at the theatre and closing the restaurant, Rudeau woke filled with the overwhelming dread along with the physical symptoms of a panic attack. Bewildered and confused, she steadily became housebound. In 1967, her marriage broke up and she fell into deep despair. The rest was a typical story: she read Weekes' first book, contacted her in Australia, where she found unstinting support, and recovered completely.

When she finally gave up on Reich, Weekes decided to appoint a willing Rudeau as the agent for her American audiotapes and videos, in order to get them back into circulation. This was yet another informal business arrangement, but, like Turner, Rudeau could be trusted. She spoke to Weekes every day, and Rudeau and Turner also kept in touch with each other. Both were increasingly concerned about Weekes, whose physical health was impaired but whose mood was even more of a concern.

Beyond Weekes' daily unhappiness, the lack of any formal recognition for her work pained her. She had no doubt about the scale of her achievement, but the only monument to her efforts was the one in her head.

As the issue of her mental state was discussed, someone came up with the idea of nominating her for a Nobel Prize. Exactly who is not entirely clear, and it's possible Weekes suggested it herself, albeit indirectly. Whatever the provenance, Rudeau enthusiastically embraced a cause that she said consumed 'hundreds and hundreds of hours'. Like Turner, like Skene Keating, Rudeau was prepared to go a long way in the service of Dr Claire Weekes.

The challenge was to recruit someone capable of undertaking such a mission. Dr Robert DuPont was an obvious candidate, but there was a catch. After Weekes had assassinated his video project in 1983, their communication had ceased, and she had resigned from the board of the Phobia Society of America, which he had invited her to join in 1980.

DuPont's experience of Weekes as a professional was one thing. He was 'in awe of her'. However, he found her personally difficult. In retrospect, he believed Weekes became paranoid. She was, he said, 'her own worst enemy fending me off summarily. She forbade me to distribute, use or save the videos we so painstakingly produced and then she turned all the rights to her tapes over to a charlatan nobody. It was gruesome. Those videos could have been useful in extending her influence which she wanted so desperately to preserve and extend.'

Regardless of his personal disappointment, DuPont was still a passionate public advocate for Weekes' ideas. Rudeau encouraged her to write to him. Weekes no longer had an address, but with the help of her friend Doreen Powell, who worked at White Plains Hospital with Zane, tracked him down, and, on 18 November 1988, five years after the video imbroglio, DuPont received a letter from Weekes out of the blue. It struck a conciliatory note. Rudeau, she wrote, had told her he was still recommending her work, as recently as the latest Phobia Society meeting in Boston. She offered no apology for the aborted video venture but said she was 'pleased and relieved that there is no ill feeling between us. I don't want any ill feeling at my age, and you were always so helpful to me.'

Weekes slid easily back into nostalgia for an intimacy that had long ago withered. She expressed her sorrow that she was 'away from you all' — a warm insinuation, and possibly a genuine expression of her isolation in Sydney. 'I had a serious head injury from a fall in the street last year which has made writing difficult, walking any distance impossible. The last two years, since then, have been difficult.' She concluded her letter saying that his recognition of her work 'has bought peace after the turmoil of the chemical imbalance vogue. Tablets used briefly can help but they can also hinder and destroy. My teaching is a safety net to catch those who fall.'

DuPont was pleased with the renewed contact, but he had

a second agenda. Her audio and video publications were useful professional resources, and he had been frustrated in attempts to obtain copies of them — including the BBC video — which were all managed by Steven Reich. Moreover, DuPont still bitterly regretted the destruction of the video they made together.

He asked his executive assistant, Patti Carson, to make enquiries with Rudeau about the availability and cost of the existing videos and the fate of his own recording. In the meantime, he wrote back to Weekes with warmth. 'Thanks for your letter. I am greatly honoured and just plain delighted to get it.' He had recommended her books highly 'because I have been so impressed by your helping so many people'.

After the initial courtesies, DuPont asked Weekes directly about the video they made together. He still hoped it could be salvaged but had no idea of its whereabouts as 'it was shipped off to you without anyone seeing it'. As for her other audio and video tapes, like everyone else in the US who tried to buy them, he had been frustrated and unable to find a source. He told her that White Plains had directed him to Rudeau in St Petersburg, Florida, to order a set and provide 'information for other people who might want them'.

He also had a professional question. While Weekes was deploring the chemical-imbalance theory, which invited drug treatment, DuPont wanted to know what she thought about combining her form of treatment 'with antidepressants and anti-anxiety medicines. Do you find the medicines help or hurt in the recovery process?'

Weekes replied in detail in a later letter, but, in between Weekes' first and second letter to DuPont, Rudeau had written to the Nobel Committee for Physiology or Medicine, in Stockholm, Sweden, asking for a copy of the nomination forms. Neither Weekes nor Rudeau mentioned the Nobel Prize to DuPont at that point, and Weekes later explained it was because she had no knowledge of it when she first wrote to him.

When Rudeau received DuPont's request for the audio and videocassettes, she simply thanked him 'for your recent letter regarding Dr Claire Weekes' tapes', sent copies of the tapes, and gave him prices. She apologised that she did not have a copy of the videotape that he had made with Weekes, but said she would look into it.

On 3 January 1989, Rudeau received confirmation from Anita Lundmark, secretary of the Nobel Committee, that her request for nomination forms had been received. On 18 January, Rudeau made her first direct approach to DuPont. Through Patti Carson, she sought DuPont's 'help/advice/opinion about nominating Dr Weekes for the Nobel Prize', adding that she had the forms from Sweden. Would DuPont like to look over the forms and help promote Weekes' candidacy? 'It would be an acknowledgement of her lifelong work and the fact that she is known worldwide,' Rudeau wrote.

Finally, Rudeau added that she had done some 'detective work' about the fate of the videotape DuPont so keenly sought. It turned out to be 'in the hands of Steve [Reich]', and the news was not good. 'He and Dr Weekes parted most acrimoniously and there is no way at this time that that tape can be obtained.' Furthermore, she added Dr Weekes had been very ill.

Although DuPont had lost his chance to recover the video, he was more than happy to help with the Nobel Prize mission, jumping in with trademark enthusiasm. Like Rudeau, he put countless hours of work into a cause he later described as quixotic. He knew how desperate Weekes was for an honour. His own opinion was that the huge grateful public response to her work spoke for itself. As someone who knew the depressing limitations of his profession, DuPont was surprised she cared for its approval at all.

A few days later, he received a long letter back from Weekes, and her communication was uncharacteristically intimate, almost pleading. At this point, she was aware he had been asked by Rudeau to help with the Nobel nomination, but unaware he had committed to it. She wanted his support, and what she said did not speak well of her life post-Coleman. Such was her state of mind that self-pity — against which she so briskly counselled in her books — was unashamedly on display for DuPont.

Yet before she listed her tribulations, she addressed the professional question she knew he wanted answered about medicating anxious patients. She diplomatically expressed delight that he was 'interested in using tranquilizers and/or antidepressants together with my teaching'. However, she was sceptical of what she called the 'adjusting chemical balance' trend in psychiatry. The idea that a chemical balance in the brain required drugs was simplistic, and her experience was that they were not particularly effective.

'Many people have been told by their therapists that this was their trouble and they have been treated accordingly.' She explained how she had received letters from people in the US saying they 'have been treated for long periods with drugs to no effect'. She added that, in Australia, the craze of 'chemical imbalance is also rife'.

This idea was now so popular that she was 'tempted to write about it as I have had quite a bit of experience with it. This subject needs an experienced view and particularly now. But I don't think I have the strength any more. I have plenty of motivation these days but the body says, "wait another day!"'

She remained open-minded about one set of drugs — sedatives. 'Of course, tranquilizers can be used with my work. For some patients. I mentioned this in my books and BBC video. Here again I could write a book on their use. I'm slightly amused at the rush for antidepressants and the rush for diagnosing depression.

Another book! But all too late!'

Then she cut to the chase. She didn't say it in so many words, but she expressed her concern that DuPont might have felt manipulated into supporting the nomination for the Nobel. When she first wrote to him, she insisted, she had no idea of Rudeau's plans, and had been 'bowled over' when she found out. Her first letter, she said, was in response to his endorsement of her work at the Phobia Society, which had inspired her to write to him 'immediately'. Yet Weekes did admit to pointing Rudeau in DuPont's direction and reminded him that he had been the first to suggest she deserved a Nobel years before.

'I remembered what you said on the same subject … in Jean Easterbrook's living room. Do you remember? I told Charlotte this and she said "I should talk to Dr DuPont about it!" I'm telling you this because I don't want you to think that was why I wrote to you. The circumstances are very strangely coincidental, but they are really coincidental.'

Then Weekes told him in detail of her poor health. There was a direct tug at his sympathy: 'it's a strange feeling facing death after a busy life thinking mainly of people and helping them. I have been so absorbed in this that death seems quite out of place — no time for it!'

Weekes also offered her own story of nervous illness, which she knew interested him. She was never agoraphobic herself, but she had had a 'debilitating illness'. She told DuPont about the sanatorium, her panic over the palpitations, the whole story — including Aurousseau.

She had been 'going over my past experiences and cannot remember any established phobia. Plenty of fear and apprehension, but no phobia.' However, she could 'well understand how one could have started. I suppose that is why I understand as you say "so well".'

Then she threw open the curtains. 'I certainly know what it's like to be nervously exhausted, right to the baseline! Especially during the last 10 years. My life has been very demanding, and I have never refused help to any patient. You should have heard my telephone during the last 30 years. It's still going — especially from the USA.'

Her final words gave a poignant insight into her changed circumstances. Reflecting on her 'especially almost impossible' last decade, Weekes set out her circumstances. 'First my well-loved sister developed Alzheimer's disease 10 years ago. She lived with me for seven of those years and often I had to look after her by myself. Finally, I had to hospitalise my brother who has a cerebral tumour, terminal. He also lived with me and is now in hospital.'

The letter had been typed out, but, in a miserable postscript, she scrawled in her tiny tense handwriting, 'during those years I almost let my sister use my brain. I don't know how I survived.'

Chapter 33

THE NOBEL NOMINATION

If Weekes was depressed, and there were some who loved her who believed that she was, it was also true that the thrill of the Nobel quest invigorated her.

In early 1989, completely fed up with Reich's inertia and frustrated that she could no longer contact him, she decided to formally shift the business to Rudeau, who was already handling it in any case. She offered Rudeau a legal contract to take over the sales and distribution of her audio and video tapes in the US. This was signed on 30 March 1989. She divided the net profits from any sales down the middle. They would get half each.

On hearing DuPont would support the Nobel Prize nomination, Weekes wrote back to him on 31 January in high excitement. 'When Charlotte told me you were willing to move toward the N.P for me (I can't even write it!) I felt happy because I know that no other person has such appreciation or knowledge of what my work has done worldwide as you! Indeed, over the past few years its influence has grown almost like a tidal wave.'

This was the first of a small wave of letters, full of exclamation marks, that DuPont received from Weekes. She knew it would fall to him to do the hard lifting, rustle up her supporters, and write the

nomination, and so she pressed upon him the scale of her achievement, divulging that, at 86, even with bouts of angina, she took at
least one call a day from individuals with particular difficulties.

> Bob, I have saved so many from leucotomy [lobotomy]
> —just on the telephone. This does not mean one or two
> calls. It may take months and I have done this, sometimes
> talking daily to the one person. I have two patients at the
> moment. I have spoken by telephone at least every second
> day to one of them. She has had the most difficult kind of
> illness to cope with — that is why have stuck to her for 18
> months. I still help even when I have had angina attacks
> (these have come with my post-operative recovery).

In the margin she added in her tiny handwriting: 'I have
charged nothing.'

Her books were 'like transfusions of hope and as such were
quickly recognised by the people — that's why they became
perennial bestsellers, and still sell surprisingly well. When I went
on TV and radio (400 times while in my 60s, 70s and 80s), you
could almost hear the sighs of relief that came over the air.'

And, 'Bob you would be surprised how many write and say I
have saved their sanity or saved them from suicide. Bob I doubt if
any doctor has done as much as I have to help nervously ill people
over the last 25 years ... And 99% of that for no financial reward!'[1]

It was one thing to sound her own trumpet, but DuPont
needed to marshal the evidence for the nomination, yet Weekes
was uncharacteristically vague. Given her age and the recent head
injury, she struggled to remember career highlights.

There had been at least one further small stroke after her fall.
Her niece Penny recalls the afternoon when, visiting Brian and
Esther at their home in the Blue Mountains, they all woke from

an afternoon nap and found Weekes had difficulty talking. In response to Penny's concern, Weekes said she was fine. 'It is just the eratreemic trashu.' She meant 'atmospheric pressure'.

Therein lay the problem for DuPont, and the nomination. DuPont tried to jog her memory. Had she written many articles, or serious papers? Were there other professionals who could endorse her?

Weekes only remembered the insult from Wolpe and struggled to think of any endorsements. There was the foremost British anxiety expert, Dr Isaac Marks in England: 'he has noted my work for years, but he is a quiet sort of bloke and I haven't a clue about whether he would help you or not'. She admitted to not being all that interested in the names of psychiatrists she met, although she 'remembered faces'.

She told him her work was taught in many of the 'National Health Clinics throughout England. It is used by the nationwide mental health association, called MIND I think. I could go on and on. After all it's been going for 25 years now Bob.' She nominated a Dr Cobb from the Priory Hospital, Roehampton, in South West London, which she said had used her work for a long time. She told DuPont her name was 'almost a household word' in England and that most clinicians knew of her.

There was Gavin Andrews in Australia, at least. He was one of the most well-known psychiatrists in Australia, running 'our best-known anxiety clinic', and she had hopes of his support.

Then there was the British psychiatrist Dr Michael Gelder, co-author of the *Oxford Textbook of Psychiatry*, who, Weekes claimed, had once said, 'Who is this woman? My patients hold her book before my eyes!' (Twenty-five years after her death, Gelder could not remember this but offered a modest endorsement: 'I remember the name Claire Weekes and I recall thinking well of her work.')

The Agoraphobic Foundation of Canada had used her work,

Weekes recalled, and she told DuPont she had been invited to address many meetings of psychiatrists at Oxford University, and hospitals in Liverpool, Cardiff, and Bradford. She listed the number of times her books were in the bestseller lists, how often they were translated, and the more serious publications that invited her to contribute.

There were unanticipated successes as well, and Weekes pointed out that after *Hope and Help for Your Nerves* was condensed by *Reader's Digest*, she had received 'letters from soldiers in Vietnam and also from USA prisons. One prisoner said he would never be in prison again because he had committed his crime while drunk and that had been because of his "nerves" which I had now cured.'

Weekes herself understood the 'difficult situation' that DuPont faced. 'I certainly do have a sparsity of publications in scientific journals (only two).' She explained she had decided against writing dignified scientific articles in favour of speaking directly to the public. 'Their need was so urgent, that I chose to write books.'

She was also grateful.

> Anyway, you don't want to hear all of this. I just wanted you to know the kind of life I have led. I know that you know so much about my pioneering effect on psychiatry today. I don't have to tell you about that. I know that you can present it as no other doctor can. That's why I'm so happy that you're doing it. Thank you, Bob. I feel those thanks as deeply as it is possible to feel thanks.

DuPont was left to round up endorsements. Zane was an obvious choice, and he immediately agreed and wrote a long letter in support of the nomination. 'What to me has been remarkable in Dr Weekes's work was her unique ability to offer invaluable understanding and advice to phobic people long before the current interest in anxieties, panic and phobias had developed and continues to do so to this day.'

As well as prominent psychiatrists, DuPont wrote to the Australian prime minister, Bob Hawke; and he knew Mel Sembler, the US ambassador to Australia, personally and contacted him. Sembler responded by saying that an endorsement from DuPont was all he needed to lend his support. 'You can certainly count on me to get her the public and professional recognition she so deserves,' Sembler reassured him. DuPont even approached Eppie Lederer, otherwise known as the popular newspaper columnist Ann Landers, who was happy to oblige.

Weekes continued to stress that she had been isolated by the profession, something DuPont did not need to be told. It was Zane whose supporting letter for the nomination asserted that 'we must also recognise and appreciate Dr Weekes's courage in pursuing her course despite the antagonistic climate of the time, and in continuing to make observations and to develop her ideas and method of treatment'.

Gavin Andrews immediately agreed to offer support. He had already thrilled Weekes by inviting her to visit his clinic earlier in the year, 'so we can honour you'. In May, he provided DuPont a supporting letter:

> Exactly as Dr DuPont says, while the rest of the professionals were trying to sedate patients, Dr Weekes was writing books and talking by telephone with countless sufferers from phobia and other forms of nervous tension. I believe that she was the first person to develop psychological techniques to enable patients to control and survive their panic attacks.
>
> In this clinic for anxiety disorders I constantly hear how the advice from Dr Weekes's books have enabled

people to survive their attacks of anxiety. Thanks to her example and now in Australia many clinics specialise in teaching people how to manage anxiety by psychological means.

DuPont's nomination letter attempted to slip across the barrier that research scientists were usually recipients of the Nobel Prize. In seven pages of advocacy, he identified anxiety as 'truly the most common, the most crippling, and the most treatable of all mental disorders'. He explained the Weekes approach and why it was superior to what was on offer elsewhere, as well as his own credentials in the field. Finally, DuPont argued that, while she had been the agent of change in the treatment of anxiety, her achievement had never been acknowledged.

> Behind and underpinning all these critical developments is the absolutely unique and timeless contributions of Dr Weekes, the retired general practitioner from Sydney, who went around the sceptical medical and psychiatric establishment and with her writing took her message of hope directly to people suffering from anxiety disorders. It is a fitting tribute to her contributions that many physicians now working with anxiety disorders, including myself, found their way to this field through patients who, in their suffering, had discovered Dr Weekes' books. In this way we found the new successful approach to the treatment of anxiety disorders.

He showed the draft Nobel nomination letter to Weekes, who typically offered some editing suggestions. She was keen that DuPont identify her criticism of the chemical-imbalance theory of nervous illness, and the drugs used to address it. 'My teaching states the opposite. I say first cure the illness and the chemical imbalance will adjust itself.'

She wanted him to stress her being a pioneer a little more strongly, and she asked if he could adjust her treatment haiku by adding two extra words, to become 'facing, accepting and floating (*not fighting*) and letting time pass'.

At the end of this letter, she acknowledged his efforts on her behalf. 'At least you know that if nothing comes of it, you have bought me a feeling of peace from a job well done and a job recognised to have been well done.'

When Rudeau wrote to DuPont on 3 April 1989 thanking him for his 'outstanding letter' in support of the nomination, she also asked him if he would 'approach the Queen, explain what we are doing and ask if she will recommend Dr Weekes for her phenomenal contribution in the field of anxiety disorders'. Not much came of that suggestion.

Ultimately, pursuit of the prize was a double-edged sword — Weekes understood the nervous system precisely because she herself was easily aroused. Rudeau wrote that, after speaking to Weekes in the evening, 'she told me how very pleased she is with your letter. In fact, during the conversation she was so excited that just talking about it made her blood pressure rise alarmingly to the point that she had to hang up the phone.' Yet Rudeau knew that happy arousal beat the alternative. 'Truly, Dr DuPont, I believe just the thought of the nomination is keeping Dr Weekes alive. I thank you for everything.'

DuPont sent his final nomination letter through for Weekes to check.

This was to be the last year of work for Weekes. She completed her final book, *The Latest Help for Your Nerves*, in May, and it was published that year. It was her least demanding book, being a compendium of articles, speeches, letters, and interviews. There was an unending appetite, it seemed, for Weekes' views on any aspect of life and how to live it. *Self Help for Your Nerves* was now in its 23rd edition.

The same year, Weekes finally received some serious recognition, when she was invited to contribute to a book on anxiety with some of the biggest names in the profession. British psychologist Roger Baker edited *Panic Disorder: theory, research, and therapy*, which also included chapters by Isaac Marks and David Barlow. Baker invited Weekes to write a joint chapter on 'the key to resisting relapse in panic', which she agreed to do. He introduced her as 'a woman ahead of her time'.

There was a personal link, as always. Roger Baker wrote of his professional debt to Weekes' work, adding that it had also helped him manage his own anxiety. 'Her way of communicating directly with patients inspired me when I was preparing a self-help book for panic written from the perspective of a clinical psychologist rather than a GP. It was published by Lion publishing in 1995 and new editions brought out in 2003 and 2011 and has been published in 13 languages. In the last chapter I emphasise the importance of Claire's approach to resisting relapse and how it was of great help to me personally in overcoming panic.'[2]

On 9 August, DuPont received a response from the secretary of the Nobel Committee that warned 'the mechanisms to invite nominators for the Nobel Prize in Physiology or Medicine are governed by rules which are very precise'. A few weeks later, DuPont and Rudeau received the news that their nomination had not made the cut.

Weekes put on a brave front. 'The news didn't surprise me,' she wrote graciously to DuPont on 19 October 1989.

> … as I said what matters is the encouragement and recognition that you and Manuel [Zane] have given me!

You made a stupendous effort with Charlotte which, in brief, helped me so much at a time when I was rather low trying to recover from the accident. Your letter was a masterpiece and to me in a sense that was my Nobel Prize, and I thank you with all my heart.

It was extremely disappointing, but 1989 was to get worse. Reich finally re-emerged, having ignored her increasingly intense overtures for the last few years. He had discovered that Rudeau had gone into business with Weekes and was selling her audios and videos in the US. Just as he had done with Yianitsas, Reich turned up on Rudeau's doorstep in Florida. He asserted his prior exclusive contractual rights to sell Weekes' audios and videos in the US. But what terrified Rudeau was that he was bearing a gun.

Turner bemoaned the fact Weekes had signed a contract with Reich that was 'in perpetuity to him'. As a result, no one else could have it during his lifetime. 'Well, he scared the living daylights out of Charlotte by the sound of it,' she wrote in a letter to Frances.

Rudeau knew Weekes wanted her, not Reich, to run the US end of the business and she had a contract to prove it. But Reich had his own contract, and a frightened Rudeau complied with his wishes, agreeing to hand over the master tapes as he had demanded. Then she asked her lawyer to write to him.

'This letter will serve as notice that Ms Rudeau will cease from advertising and selling. Further the master tapes have been returned to you. Ms Rudeau does not wish to be contacted again by yourself by mail or phone. Please do not threaten Ms Rudeau any more as that will just complicate matters.'

Although Reich would have been deeply indifferent, the lawyer threw in that 'Ms Rudeau has given thousands of hours of her time freely and with dedication to Dr Weekes' work and feels unjustly used in this entire procedure.'

None of this improved Weekes' mood. There was no Nobel, her work was back in the inert hands of an impossible individual who had let her down quite personally, Rudeau was distressed, and now Weekes was left with only the impositions of an ageing body and an unsatisfactory life.

DuPont's executive assistant, Patti Carson, wrote to him saying that Weekes was 'really very down when she didn't get the Nobel prize, even though she didn't really expect it'. The woman who knew about depletion, who understood exactly how physical illness could lead to mental disturbances, was depressed. That was her friends' diagnosis.

Weekes herself had so often pointed out that real grief was felt in the two organs that respond so sympathetically — the heart and the gut — and hers were now in genuine strife. At the age of 86, her body was letting her down, as were a number of people, and she was struggling with the known consequences.

Chapter 34

FINAL DAYS

Not long after the Nobel nomination was rejected, Weekes asked an extraordinary favour of Rudeau. Could she come to live with her in St Petersburg, Florida? It was a remarkable request from an elderly woman with health problems and an extended family in Australia but said everything about her state of mind. Weekes wanted a new life. Among other concerns, she dreaded a fate like that of her remaining siblings, who were in institutional care.

There is no record of how Rudeau responded to the proposition, but Weekes stayed in Australia. The two women talked every day on the phone in this bleak period. Patti Carson captured the miserable uncertainty of Weekes' existence, writing that 'for a while Dr Weekes wanted to come to live with Charlotte to promote the work, but that seems to have passed. There are major problems in Dr Weekes' family and they talked about putting her in a nursing home.'

Weekes life was now beyond her control. She wanted to run away, but that option was unrealistic, and she was left in Sydney with a divided family, under stress. Without Coleman to shield her, Weekes had faced more chaos in the last ten years of her life than in the previous seven decades.

Closer to 90 than 80, she regularly referred to her 'old ticker' and continued to battle blood pressure. She knew her health was precarious but resisted any attempt to get her to see a heart specialist. Weekes didn't want to know too much, and, in any case, she treated herself. Yet she hated rows, fuss, and drama, and, in the face of family pressures, she dithered.

Rudeau decided to make a further effort to secure a Nobel nomination. She enlisted a 'supporting group' who would round up some Nobel Laureates directly, particularly the latest winners for medicine.

More realistically, Rudeau also initiated a nomination for the Order of Australia. DuPont was happy to support this. The work had already been done for the Nobel, so they just reassembled it for the Australian award.

Beyond the problems with her health, her family, and Reich, there was now a dreadful new shadow, one that was all too real, and intractable to her techniques. Her respectable, leafy neighbourhood, with its large homes and quiet wealth and privilege, was being stalked by a murderer. Dubbed the 'granny killer', he preyed on elderly women living alone. He had murdered his first victim in March 1989, in Mosman, her adjoining suburb. By May, it was obvious a serial killer was on the rampage.

The murders all took place in the same corner of Sydney, and Weekes took the threat seriously. Elderly women were being either bludgeoned or strangled by a man who followed them home. He only struck on weekdays, when the women were most likely to be alone. The sensational details were given wide publicity, compounding the fear. Weekes told her Dial an Angel companion Pat Ryder that she didn't feel safe at night.

On 3 November, Brian died. Dulcie passed away exactly three weeks later, on 24 November. Weekes was the eldest of her siblings and had survived them all. Most of her generation, barring her great friend Cecily Aurousseau and her sister-in-law Esther, were gone.

With Dulcie's death, the fate of the house was another spectre to haunt Weekes. She had never organised her final security over the property. Her own tenancy could well be precarious, depending on the attitude of Dulcie's beneficiaries. While there was no suggestion that her nieces would put it on the market while she was alive, Weekes no longer had assured authority over her living arrangements.

She had a great horror of ending up in institutionalised care, but, by late 1989, she was unhappy and frightened in her own home. By December, her misery was apparent among the wider family, and her eldest niece, Frances, offered to have her in Canberra for a few weeks. This stay extended to four months. Weekes would never return to 37 Milson Road. She left all her possessions behind and bid goodbye to Pat Ryder, saying, 'It is better for me to go to Canberra. I can't stand it here anymore after all the good years I have had.'

A measure of her desperation to leave was her destination. From a residence with what her nieces describe as 'mansion' dimensions, she had moved to a spartan Canberra home. 'It must have been a huge upheaval,' says Frances, 'as, at the time, I only had a small government house at Page [a suburb in the outer ring of Canberra]. No magnificent view, and a very small garden.'

Worse still, Australia's capital was a well-planned government city, its earnestness alleviated by a topography that was beautiful, but it was not Sydney Harbour. Sprawling suburbs sat in an undulating landscape, ringed by forested mountains. It was known as the Bush Capital, and the newer suburbs looked as if they had been plonked on a sheep run. Canberra was a very mixed blessing. Weekes felt safe there, and the city was nothing if not peaceful, yet she loved company and here there were trees but no people. Beyond the city centre, Australia's capital city was dead by day. Frances worked full-time and, when Weekes was lonely, she rang her niece at work, which did not endear Frances to her boss.

The blood clot on the brain, high blood pressure, and relentless digestive problems made daily life a trial. Her mind remained acute, but there were malapropisms, a legacy of the aneurysm. Compact discs became 'compound discs'. Frances recalls the 'asparagus to seeing the stars', which she later discerned was a reference to her binoculars. Weekes had meant to say 'apparatus'. Despite the quirks of speech, Weekes remained a fine singer, capable of beautiful renditions of German lieder.

There was another legacy, apparently, and the first Frances heard of it was when one day she danced through the house, swirling her skirt, to be met with the remark, 'You come from a long line of masculine women, luvvie.' Frances assumed when her aunt selected the word 'masculine', she meant trailblazer. That was certainly how Weekes saw herself.

As her 87-year-old aunt was still mobile, Frances could take her out to restaurants and movies. One day at lunch with Frances and her daughter and son-in-law, Weekes observed that she was happy 'because she felt loved'.

Steven Reich remained a headache to the last. DuPont wanted to press ahead with the lawsuit against him, and planned to persuade Weekes to use her Sydney lawyer to threaten Reich with legal action unless he permitted Weekes to distribute her materials 'as she sees fit in the future' — or 'we will get him for nonperformance for the last three years'. The fallback position was to negotiate the most favourable financial deal possible, to ensure that the material remained publicly available.

At first, Weekes agreed to the legal action, but it was not long before she backed off. Rudeau wrote to DuPont explaining that 'presented with the options, Weekes had chosen to write Steve personally, appealing for his cooperation'. Rudeau then added with what seemed like extraordinary optimism that 'she is expecting a call from him that all will be well'.

On 11 January 1990, Weekes wrote an ingratiating letter to

Reich. She explained her new living circumstances, gave him her telephone number, and made a muted appeal to his honour: 'As you know I have practically lived for my work, and having entrusted to you the promotion and distribution of my cassettes and videos in the USA, I would like, therefore, to help you as much as possible.' She wanted to know Reich's plans for promotion and distribution — she had some ideas of her own, she said, which she would 'like to submit for your approval'. This incorrigible individual, who had sat on her work, and refused to either share it with anyone else or even explain himself to her, was again being humoured.

It didn't work. In March, Rudeau updated DuPont. Weekes, she said, was 'frustrated, angry'. Reich had virtually buried her work. 'All enquiries, orders from clients for tapes are directed to Steven Reich, who is not responding to them. Five months have passed, people call me to complain that their letters go unanswered, and no one can do a thing. Her attorney continues to tell her to give him more time, but her patience is running out.'

In April, Weekes tried again, although her letter sounded defeated. 'Apparently you are not answering requests sent to box 867. I'm sure if you and I could communicate amicably we could save Worth Productions to our mutual advantage.'

Ratcheting up the pressure, she tackled Reich directly for the first time.

'You have never even told me how many records, cassettes or videos we have sold or hired out during the last 13 years. I asked [attorney] Stephen Bodzin several times during those years to ask you to give me a reckoning, but you never sent me one.'

Weekes wondered if he was 'frightened', perhaps because she had asked an accountant's assessment of Worth Production's finances since 1977 (debt and credit) and because he 'may not have kept any books for Worth Productions during those years. If this is so, would you just send me a simple list of debts and credits, and, when I check it, if I'm satisfied with this, I will pay what I owe. I am no longer asking for an accountant's assessment. I would accept a bona fide list from you but not just a telephoned statement. I want to pay any debts before I die. I can only hope you answer this.'

It was hard to imagine there were any debts from the business, but perhaps Weekes offered this as bait. He didn't take it. She never heard from Reich again.

In March 1990, the 'granny killer' was caught and arrested. John Glover, an Englishman in his late 50s with a wife and two daughters and a job as a pie salesman, was sentenced to life imprisonment in November 1991. After a bout of cancer, he took his own life in jail in 2005.

Not long after Glover's arrest, Frances returned home from work to be told that her aunt had decided to leave Canberra and return to Sydney. Frances had employed two women to come in during the day to keep her aunt company, but Weekes was missing Sydney. She had decided to sell her home, telling Frances she could not bear to go back. Also, 'there are too many memories there for me now. Mum, Dulcie and Beth.'

Without telling Frances, Weekes had negotiated a move to the retirement home in Warriewood where Esther lived. She had asked her lawyers to help her sort this out. She organised the sale of the house in Cremorne and made arrangements to parcel off most of her possessions. The licensed conveyancer at a Northern Beaches legal practice, Ann Blannin-Ferguson, was privy to some of Weekes' concerns about her life. She particularly remembers Weekes saying that she wished Coleman was around to help with decisions.

The decision to move into institutional care must have been hard, yet Frances says her aunt was 'amazingly calm about the whole situation'. On 11 April, Weekes turned 87. 'You can live too long', she told Frances once when tired and unhappy. While still in Canberra, she had told a visiting friend from Melbourne that she was ready to die, and that her last year had been troubled.

For a short time before she finally moved into the retirement home, Weekes stayed with Cecily Aurousseau. All through this period, Weekes kept up daily conversations with Rudeau, who reported to DuPont that her mood had improved. She was 'wonderfully feisty. It was "on with the Nobel, on with the Order of Australia, on with the work."'

The lawyers helped to organise respite care in an apartment near Esther, as well as the payment of $95,000 for permanent residency. Perhaps the restful presence and companionship of Esther — her own age, her own family — offered some consolation for the prospect of institutional life. A friend later wrote to Esther that she had telephoned Weekes on her second day in the retirement home and found her 'well and cheerful, and she told me what a wonderful welcome you had given her'.

So, there they were, two old women, tied together by the bonds of family, affection, and memories. Weekes was a diminished figure. Her great-nephew Adam, who had revelled in his special childish place in the 'Beth and Claire' firmament, saw how her great spirit had flagged. As a teenager, Adam had visited his grandmother Dulcie in her nursing home, and, although he was busy, the 19-year-old made time to catch up with Aunty Claire not long after she arrived in Warriewood. He noticed the change in her immediately, and found it affecting. 'She was physically frail, thin, shaky, and weak. And it was tough to see her that way because she was always such a pillar of strength in the family.'

Not long after, on 2 June 1990, Weekes had another visitor, her niece Tita. Tita hated the idea that her aunt was locked into an aged-care facility instead of living out her days overlooking Sydney Harbour. Knowing an institution was the last place Weekes had ever wanted to find herself, Tita decided to visit her there. It had been a long time since they had spoken, and Tita was not entirely well, feeling shaky and emotional. Recounting the experience almost 30 years later, the words tumble out.

'I knocked on the door and she was surprised, but happy to see me. I don't think I looked too good at the time because there was still so much going on and I was very stressed.'

She told her aunt she had come to give her 'a really huge thank-you for everything you have done for us: for taking us in and giving us a roof over our heads, loving us, having such a generous spirit, and being so positive about all of us, all of the time. I'm dreadfully sorry for whatever happened that hurt you because we've both been hurt, and I just want you to know I love you, more than anything. You and Mum. You have been so fantastic, and I just wanted to tell you that.'

According to Tita, Weekes responded by hugging her. She looked happy, but what she said next just hung in the air, unexplained. 'I've made a terrible mistake,' her aunt said.

In the intensity of the moment, Tita did not ask, and her aunt said no more. It was a short meeting, and Tita was not long home when the news came through. Weekes had been found dead in front of her dressing-room table in her small apartment. She had been about to do her hair in preparation for the communal meal. She had been in the retirement village for less than a week.

It was a swift passing. 'I have rarely attended a person actually dying that realised that he, or she, was dying', wrote Weekes in her penultimate book, six years earlier. 'Nature blunts the edge of her sword.'[1] The heart that had taught her about anxiety in her 20s had beaten on for another six decades.

Esther was left $50,000, to be passed on to her two children, Timothy and Barbara, on her death. Penny was left $25,000. The rest of the estate was divided equally between Frances, Lili, and Tita. This included ongoing copyright payments for the books, audio, and video. The value of the whole estate, including the proceeds from the house at Cremorne, was just over $1.4 million. For a woman whose bestselling books had made so much money over the years, this was not great wealth. Nothing about Weekes' finances would ever be simple. Her will would later be challenged, successfully, by Penny, and the legal complications of her unresolved business relationships would continue for decades.

On 18 June 1990, the US ambassador, Mel Sembler, wrote a letter to D.I. Smith, the secretary of the Order of Australia. The ambassador sought to 'strongly support the nomination' of Dr Claire Weekes, one of Australia's most distinguished citizens, for an appointment to the Order of Australia.

> Dr Weekes has been a pioneer for decades in the treatment of phobias and anxieties and through her innovative methods and her publications, she has helped millions of phobic sufferers all over the world to recover from their debilitating conditions and lead full and productive lives once again. It has been estimated that half of those who have benefited from her work have been Americans. Dr Weekes is not only revered by those she has helped, but she is beloved by her colleagues in the United States as well. As the representative of so many of my countrymen whose lives of been touched by her, I am pleased to commend her to you.

Four days later, Sembler again wrote to his friend Bob DuPont in Washington.

> Dear Bob,
>
> Sitting atop my desk awaiting a signature upon my return from the US was the enclosed letter seconding

the nomination of Dr Claire Weekes for the Order of Australia. Sadly, just as I was ready to sign the letter came the news of Dr Weekes' death. The Secretariat of the Order has informed us that they do not award posthumous honours. Fortunately, so many people have been helped by Dr Weekes that her work will live on.

Epilogue

WHAT LIVES ON

I meet Saeed Fassaie on a blustery summer afternoon outside a suburban Sydney library, and we walk to a local cafe, where he tells me his story of a woman we have in common.

An Iranian immigrant to Australia, Fassaie has recently published his memoir, *Rising from the Shadows*.[1] It's the story of his life, and his breakdown, as well as his recovery. Fassaie migrated to Australia in 1998, after serving in the war between Iran and Iraq. There, his best friend, Darius, had been shot, and Fassaie had been witness to his mutilated body.

One night, about a decade later, in a safe, leafy Sydney suburb, Fassaie watched a film set in France during World War II. He found himself unexpectedly agitated, his heart racing uncontrollably, and went to bed in a distressed state, flooded by intrusive memories of his friend's dead body. On waking, there was no improvement, and he feared a heart attack. Ashamed of his reaction, Fassaie didn't mention his frightening symptoms to his family, and instead, after dinner in the evenings, he would travel to the local Chatswood library in search of enlightenment from the self-help section.

He read every book that seemed vaguely relevant. 'Not only did they not help, they made me feel worse,' he recalls. He saw psychologists. One just wanted to talk about the Iran–Iraq War; the other seemed obsessed with money. He gave up on them.

One night, moving from the self-help section to the health section, Fassaie happened to pick up a book by Dr Claire Weekes, 'who described my symptoms so perfectly I felt she was using me as a case study. At last, I had found someone who could understand me! It was astounding. I borrowed the book and continued reading it through the night until I literally couldn't keep my eyes open. This was a breakthrough.'

The words on those pages had been written almost 40 years before, yet were still in print, still available in bookshops and libraries around the world.

Twenty-five years after Weekes' death, Fassaie published his autobiography, recounting a life that the now-successful structural engineer considers fortunate. The subtitle is *revolution, war, and the journey that made me.*

The dedication on the front page is to a woman he never met:

> To the memory of Dr Claire Weekes, the late Australian mental health writer and physician. You live on through the lives of the countless sufferers your works continue to help. I humbly thank you for penning some of the most insightful and liberating lines I have ever read.

Acknowledgements

———————

Without a publisher, there is no book. My deep thanks go to Henry Rosenbloom, publisher of Scribe, for his confidence in the story I wanted to tell and for letting me get on with it. With Scribe came the fastidious editor David Golding, who I thank for so ably and sympathetically helping me clear a path to the destination.

When I first considered writing about Dr Claire Weekes, I assumed her story had been told and was astonished to find the field wide open. While her ideas appeared as useful as ever — and her books were still on sale — Weekes herself had come and gone.

My first tentative enquiry into the prospect of a biography drew an immediate email response from Dr Robert DuPont, a Washington-based psychiatrist.

How can I help you?

Dr Weekes had a profound, positive influence on my life and my work in anxiety disorders — and the field itself. But no one but you and I know that. Maybe your book can change that.

Bob's unstinting support sits like a foundation beneath the book. I also benefited from the cooperation of his two daughters, Elizabeth DuPont Spencer and Caroline DuPont, both psychologists who have written books on anxiety. The DuPont family was a lighthouse across the Pacific, and I can't thank them enough.

The support of the Weekes family was indispensable, and I am so very grateful to them all in different and important ways. They are a family of great conversationalists, and Weekes crackled alive for me from their varied versions until I felt I was leading a parallel life.

Frances Maclaren supplied documents and measureless time, patiently assisting my excavations of her aunt's and the family's past. Penny Weekes, Tita Blaiklock, Adam Blaiklock, Lili Louez, Barbara Preyssass, Tim Weekes, Christina Stephen, David Weekes, and Nick Coles offered their recollections, and some endured ongoing interrogation, particularly Penny.

I never left Penny's company without another book on the mind or brain, and Tita provided the wonderful photo for the front cover, along with letters and frank, fascinating recollections. Barbara's great memory and her father's memoirs were a blessing. Lili and Adam could not have been more helpful. The family research was mostly great fun, but I am also indebted to them for their trust and cooperation.

I was fortunate to find Marcel Aurousseau's nephew Neville Aurousseau, who pulled into focus an uncle whose exceptional intellectual abilities were indivisible from a wry humour. My thanks for his memories and the photos of Marcel.

For Weekes' school years, I am indebted to the efforts of Gaenor Williams, the archivist at Sydney Girls High School for providing documents and photos that showed Weekes' zest for life and learning. Thanks also to Lee R. Hiltzik from the Rockefeller Archive Centre and Robert Winckworth from the UCL Records

Office for their help in providing institutional records.

To understand Weekes the scientist, I initially contacted Professor Mike Thompson, then the Deputy Dean of Science and Professor in Zoology at the University of Sydney. I was thrilled to get another immediate, enthusiastic response. Mike was most generous with his time, and from him I learned of Weekes' seminal contribution in a second specialist field. He also very kindly looked over some of the relevant chapters.

Dr Susan Jones at the University of Tasmania and Jane Thompson, a former zoologist, generously translated some of the complexities of Weekes' early work. I thank them and Dr Richard Shine, emeritus professor and zoologist at the University of Sydney, who read parts of my manuscript, directed me to relevant publications, and pointed me towards Dr Glenn Shea at the Sydney School of Veterinary Science.

My deep thanks to Dr Shea, whose assistance was invaluable as he shared his deep knowledge of Australian anatomical and zoological history along with its myriad of fascinating scholars, as well as steadying my wobbly understanding of evolutionary science. He is an exacting scholar, and some of my chapters are the better for his critical input.

As for Weekes' second career, in mental health, I found professionals willing to help because of their high regard for her work. The meticulous, insightful Dr Sally Winston, the founder and co-director of the Anxiety and Stress Disorders Institute of Maryland, was one of these. Sally assisted in clearing the clouds in my understanding of where Weekes sat in the arc of psychiatric and psychological history.

Her co-author of several books on anxiety, Dr Martin Seif, was similarly illuminating — my thanks to them both and also to Robert Ackerman for his time and memories. All three were hugely helpful and important sources of information, given their extensive exposure to the work of Weekes in the US and their enthusiasm for her approach.

Dr Winston also directed me to the pioneering work of the eminent neuroscientist Joseph LeDoux on anxiety and his epic work *Anxious*.[1] Here I saw fascinating parallels with Weekes' much earlier concepts of fear and the brain. I thank Professor LeDoux for his subsequent generosity, and his invaluable eye on a chapter pertinent to his own work. How he found the time between the academy and his band, the Amygdaloids, is a mystery, but I am immensely grateful.

I was drawn to the work of Emeritus Professor Richard Burkhardt, from the Department of History at the University of Illinois, who wrote the modern landmark study of Lamarck. He was another scholar who had never heard of Weekes yet was most generous with his fine advice, and kindly read some of my work.

To Dr David Barlow, a special mention. As he is a renowned global expert in the field, it was wonderful to have him confirm Weekes' pioneering contribution. I am grateful for the time and trouble he took responding to my questions, and grateful that he cared to so generously put his own views on the public record.

Dr Isaac Marks, now retired, but one of the UK's pre-eminent anxiety experts, alerted me to his acknowledgement of her work, and Dr Roger Baker, Professor of Clinical Psychology at Bournemouth University, helpfully directed my attention to his textbook *Panic Disorder: theory, research, and therapy*,[2] in which he had included the work of Weekes. I also thank Professor William C. Sanderson and the late Dr Michael Gelder.

I am indebted to Dr Raymond DiGiuseppe — who worked very closely with Albert Ellis — for his memories of her work, and of their recognition of her achievement in the US.

In Australia, Professor Gavin Andrews, one of Australia's pre-eminent anxiety specialists, was interviewed at length and kindly read a number of the chapters. His professional and personal observations were extremely valuable, and I am in debt to him for his assistance and support. I also thank two other Australian professionals in the field, Dr John Franklin and Professor Ron Rapee.

In the Sydney medical fraternity, I would like to thank Dr Robert Holland and Dr John York in particular.

I was fortunate enough to have a good friend, Dr Judy Proudfoot, herself a specialist in the field of anxiety, who very kindly introduced me to two colleagues at the Black Dog Institute in Australia: Dr Peter Baldwin, a research fellow, and Professor Vijaya Manicavasagar, the director of their Psychology Clinic.

Dr Baldwin offered important clarifications, and diplomatically corrected a misconception or two. I so appreciated his time, given his very tight schedule. A huge thank you to him, and, in the same measure, to Professor Manicavasagar.

I offer the standard, unarguable, disclaimer that no matter how many eyes have passed over a page, the mistakes are the author's alone.

Beyond the Weekes family, there are those who knew the woman herself and who were generous with their time and memories. I am just sorry the late Anne Turner did not live to see the biography to which she made such a significant contribution. Fran Groves, the BBC producer who worked with Weekes in the mid-1980s, was another open-hearted respondent, with her recollection of the 'colossus of calm'. I thank her for her acute observations and the helpful and enjoyable correspondence.

To Paul Skene Keating, my deep gratitude for his support for the book and his willingness to discuss his family's relationship with Weekes and Coleman with such candour and insight. I also thank him for the rare photographs of Beth.

At White Plains, Judy Chessa and the retired Doreen Powell kindly shared their memories, and Judy provided some helpful documentation. My warm thanks to them and likewise to Dr Manuel Zane's two daughters, Sharon and Carolyn, whose real effort to share their memories and to provide relevant documents I deeply appreciate, as it gave me a good understanding of this important relationship for Weekes and of Dr Zane's own exceptional professional contribution.

Richard Walsh had the benefit of knowing Dr Weekes and is renowned for generous sharing. He was another who saw the value of a biography of Weekes, and I am grateful for his assistance and enthusiasm, as well as permission to tell his personal story.

Thanks also to Craig Munro, award-winning biographer of Weekes' incorrigible literary agent Percy Reginald Stephensen. Craig offered encouragement and advice at a time it was needed and kindly advised on one or two chapters.

My thanks also to David Johnson for his time and recollections of Dr Weekes.

Many of these individuals could have been found by any biographer, but occasionally you get lucky. I was fortunate to trip across Ralph Bollweg, who helped educate me, peppering me with terrific suggestions from his encyclopaedic reading list, along with some robust opinions of mental-health professionals. Bollweg regards Weekes as an oasis of sanity in a confused and incompetent profession. I thank him for the great correspondence.

As a journalist, I am surrounded by writers. They are a generous bunch. My manuscript benefited from the astute eye and high-beam attention of my dear friend, the author and journalist Pamela Williams. Thanks, Pam, for treating an extraordinary effort as an ordinary act of friendship. It was so much more.

To those of my great friends who helped me to wrestle the book into being, a huge thank-you — Julie Flynn and Trevor Cook, Brian Toohey, Andrew Clark, Tony Walker, Andrew Cornell, and Jill Margo.

Some were spared, but for long-distance conversational endurance and excellent advice, particularly from those for whom anxiety is no more than an itch, I thank the following dear friends: Kyrsty Macdonald, Catherine Fox, Lis Sexton, Deborah Hope, Deirdre Macken, Marie and Greg Wood, Margaret and Max Bourke, Helen Trinca, and Jos Hackforth-Jones. And thanks to Philip Yates for his thoughtfulness!

To Jenny Brockie, for being there, always, with love and thanks.

And now to my family: Everyone needs a wise and wonderful sister, and I thank Cathy Hoare with love. And thanks to my dear nieces: Gillian Fahey, who helped out with transcripts, and who always has an interesting take on life; and her sister, Monica Fahey, the clever young scientist prepared to talk about evolution with her aunt. Thanks to my stepdaughter, Kate Crawford, with love, for inspiration of the non-anxious kind. Thanks to my darling daughter, Claudia Crawford, for her total support and the gift of her crisp, intelligent observations.

To the memory of my dearly loved and loving parents, Barbara and George Hoare.

Finally, thanks to my beloved husband, Jim, a true believer if ever there was one. From the very outset, he understood exactly the story I wanted to tell, and his confidence in it, and in me, was unwavering and helped make four years glide by joyously.

Notes

Claire Weekes wrote the following five books, published in Australia and the UK by Angus & Robertson:

SHFYN   *Self Help for Your Nerves*. 1962.
          (Published in the US as *Hope and Help for Your Nerves*.)

PFNS   *Peace from Nervous Suffering*. 1972.

SETOA   *Simple, Effective Treatment of Agoraphobia*. 1977.

MHFYN   *More Help for Your Nerves*. 1984.

TLHFYN   *The Latest Help for Your Nerves*. 1989.

Chapter 1. MISDIAGNOSIS

1 Vere Hole, W. & Treweeke, A.H. *The History of the Women's College within the University of Sydney*. Angus & Robertson. 1953.

Chapter 2. HER MOTHER'S DAUGHTER

1 Sherington, G. & Campbell, C. 'Education'. *Sydney Journal* 2(1). June 2009. https://epress.lib.uts.edu.au/ojs/index.php/sydney_journal/article/viewFile/886/1187
2 *The Sydney Mail*. 16 July 1881. p154.
3 Hutton Neve, M. *This Mad Folly!: the history of Australia's pioneer women doctors*. Library of Australian History. 1980.
4 ibid.

Chapter 3. THE EVOLUTION OF CLAIRE

1 *The West Australian*. 23 August 1926.
2 Walsh, G.P. in the *Australian Dictionary of Biography*.
3 ibid.
4 *The Australian Worker*. 7 March 1928.
5 Harrison, L. *The Present Position of the Evolution Problem: being the Livingstone Lectures for 1924*. Marchant & Co. 1925. p36.
6 ibid. p13.
7 ibid. p53.

Chapter 4. MEETING MARCEL

1 *The Newcastle Sun*. 9 February 1925. p6.
2 Nicholas, F.W. & Nicholas, J.M. *Charles Darwin in Australia*. Cambridge University Press. 2002. p124.
3 *The Newcastle Sun*. 23 January 1925.
4 *The Newcastle Herald*. 24 January 1925. p1.

5   Woollacott, A. *To Try Her Fortune in London: Australian women, colonialism, and modernity*. Oxford University Press. 2001.

6   *The Maitland Daily Mercury*. 17 February 1925. p4.

7   *The Newcastle Sun*. 20 January 1925. p5.

8   ibid.

9   *The Newcastle Sun*. 20 January 1925, p5 (twice); 30 January 1925, p7; 3 February 1925, p2.

10 *The Sydney Morning Herald*. 6 February 1925. p3.

11 *The Newcastle Sun*. 30 January 1925. p7.

12 *The Sun* (Sydney). 18 December 1930. p25.

13 Oral history. National Library of Australia. Recorded by Hazel de Berg, 30 June 1977.

14 ibid.

15 Varpian, T. et al. 'In Memoriam'. *Australian Geographer* 16(1). 1984. p1.

16 Bean, C. *Official History of Australia in the War of 1914–1918, vol. 3: the Australian Imperial Force in France, 1916*. Angus & Robertson. 1923. p728.

17 *The Evening News* (Sydney). 3 February 1917. p6.

18 Siers, R. & Walker, C. *Ancestry: stories of multicultural Anzacs*. Department of Veterans' Affairs. 2015. https://www.awm.gov.au/sites/default/files/Ancestry_2015.pdf

19 Oral history, op. cit.

Chapter 5. LIZARD BABIES AND THE LIZARD BRAIN

1   Hoare, M. & Rutledge, M. in the *Australian Dictionary of Biography*.

2   Harrison, L. & Weekes, H.C. 'On the Occurrence of Placentation in the Scincid Lizard *Lygosoma entrecasteauxi*'. *Proceedings of the Linnean Society of New South Wales* 50. 1925.

3   Shine, R. 'Evolution of an Evolutionary Hypothesis: a history of changing ideas about the adaptive significance of viviparity in reptiles'. *Journal of Herpetology* 48(2). June 2014. pp147–61.

4   Harrison & Weekes, op. cit.

5   *The Sun.* 24 April 1926.

6   *Table Talk.* 20 October 1927. p5.

7   *Official Year Book of the Commonwealth of Australia, no. 23: 1930.* Commonwealth Bureau of Census and Statistics. 1930. p377.

Chapter 6. THE SHADOW OF DEATH

1   *Dungog Chronicle.* 28 February 1928.

2   *The Sun.* 21 February 1928.

3   Woollacott, A. *To Try Her Fortune in London: Australian women, colonialism, and modernity.* Oxford University Press. 2001.

4   Application for Rockefeller Fellowship by Claire Weekes. Courtesy of the Rockefeller Foundation.

5   Hogben, L. *Lancelot Hogben, Scientific Humanist.* Merlin Press. 1998.

6   Dawson, W.R. (ed.) *Sir Grafton Elliot Smith: a biographical record by his colleagues.* Jonathan Cape. 1938. p186.

7   Kay, L.E. *The Molecular Vision of Life: Caltech, the Rockefeller Foundation, and the rise of the new biology.* Oxford University Press. 1996.

8   ibid.

9   Professor William Dakin, from the University of Sydney in support of Weekes' application for a Rockefeller Fellowship to the University College London.

10 Kinghorn, J.R. 'A New Species of *Lygosoma* from New South Wales'. *Proceedings of the Linnean Society of New South Wales* 54. 1929. pp32–3.

Chapter 7. SINKING AND FLOATING

1   Unknown woman calling David Johnson on his New Zealand radio program discussing the work of Dr Weekes. Radio Pacific.

2   BBC interview with Marian Foster. 1986. Reproduced in TLHFYN p46.

3   Talk given at the Fourth National Phobia Conference, Phobia and
     Anxiety Clinic, White Plains Hospital, New York. 7 May 1983.
     Reproduced in MHFYN.

4   Interview with Marian Foster, part six. *Pebble Mill at One*. BBC. 1983.

5   Letter to Robert DuPont. 15 January 1989.

6   MHFYN p35.

7   ibid.

Chapter 8. DARWIN AND THE HEART OF THE MATTER

1   Barlow, N. (ed.) *The Autobiography of Charles Darwin, 1809–1882*.
     Collins. 1958.

2   Ruse, M. 'Is Evolution a Secular Religion?' *Science* 299(5612). 7 March
     2003. p1523.

3   Pickering, G. *Creative Malady*. Oxford University Press. 1974. p34.

4   Pasnau, R.O. 'Darwin's Illness: a biopsychosocial perspective'.
     Psychosomatics 31(2). 1990. pp121–8.

5   Darwin, C. Letter 3879. Darwin Correspondence Project.
     http://www.darwinproject.ac.uk/DCP-LETT-3879

6   Ekman, P. 'Darwin's Contributions to Our Understanding of
     Emotional Expressions'. *Philosophical Transactions of the Royal Society B*
     364(1535). 12 December 2009.

7   ibid.

8   Darwin, C. *The Expression of the Emotions in Man and Animals*. John
     Murray. 1872. p12.

9   ibid.

10   Schore, A. *The Dr Drew Podcast* 65. 12 June 2013.

11   Wilson, D.S. & Hayes, S.C. *Evolution and Contextual Behavioural Science:
     an integrated framework for understanding, predicting, and influencing human
     behaviour*. Context Press. 2018.

12   Freud, S. *An Autobiographical Study*. 1925.

13 Sulloway, F. *Freud, Biologist of the Mind*. Harvard University Press. 1979. p276.

14 Freud, S. *A General Introduction to Psychoanalysis*. First delivered as lectures 1915–1917 and first translated into English in 1920.

15 Brenner, C. *An Elementary Textbook of Psychoanalysis*. Anchor Books. 1974. p70.

16 Sulloway, op. cit. p4.

17 Darwin, op. cit. p219.

18 Richardson, R.D. *William James: in the maelstrom of American modernism*. Houghton Mifflin Harcourt. 2006. p89.

19 Wilson & Hayes, op. cit.

20 James, W. *The Principles of Psychology*. Henry Holt & Co. 1890.

21 Ellsworth, P.C. 'William James and Emotion: is a century of fame worth a century of misunderstanding?' *Psychological Review* 101(2). 1994. pp222–9.

22 Cannon, W.B. *Bodily Changes in Pain, Hunger, Fear, and Rage: an account of recent researches into the function of emotional excitement*. Appleton. 1915. p211.

23 Cannon, W.B. *The Role of Emotion in Disease*. 1936.

24 Dalgleish, T. 'The Emotional Brain'. *Nature Reviews Neuroscience* 5(7). July 2004. p582.

25 Barrett, L.F. *How Emotions Are Made: the secret life of the brain*. Pan Books. 2016.

26 Tinbergen, N. *The Study of Instinct*. Oxford University Press. 1951. pp4–5.

27 LeDoux, J. *Anxious: the modern mind in the age of anxiety* (UK edition). Oneworld. 2015.

Chapter 9. NOW, HERE WAS A TEACHER

1 Oral history. National Library of Australia. Recorded by Hazel de Berg, 30 June 1977.

2   *The News* (Adelaide). 7 May 1937. p7.

3   Saito, A. *Bartlett, Culture, and Cognition*. Routledge. 2000. p33.

4   Wilson, D.S. & Hayes, S.C. *Evolution and Contextual Behavioural Science: an integrated framework for understanding, predicting, and influencing human behaviour*. Context Press. 2018.

5   Derricourt, R. 'The Australian who Rewrote World History'. *Inside Story*. 10 August 2015. https://insidestory.org.au/the-australian-who-rewrote-world-history/

6   Dawson, W.R. (ed.) *Sir Grafton Elliot Smith: a biographical record by his colleagues*. Jonathan Cape. 1938. p185.

7   Elliot Smith, G. *The Evolution of the Mind*. Royal Institution of Great Britain. 1934.

8   Dawson, op. cit.

9   Waldron, H.A. 'The Study of the Human Remains from Nubia: the contribution of Grafton Elliot Smith and his colleagues to palaeopathology'. *Medical History* 44(3). August 2000. p385.

10 *The Sydney Morning Herald*. 25 June 1914.

11 Ackerknecht, E.H. 'The History of the Discovery of the Vegetative (Autonomic) Nervous System'. *Medical History* 18(1). January 1974. pp1–8.

12 Davis, D.L. & Whitten, R.G. 'Medical and Popular Traditions of Nerves'. *Social Science and Medicine* 26(12). 1988. pp1209–21.

13 SHFYN p5.

14 Dawson, op. cit. p60.

15 ibid.

16 Elliot Smith, op. cit. p2.

Chapter 10. A TEMPLATE FOR A BOOK

1   Breger, L. *Freud: darkness in the midst of vision*. John Wiley & Sons. 2000. p260.

2   ibid.

3   ibid.

4   ibid. p242.

5   Elliot Smith, G. & Pear, T.H. *Shell Shock and Its Lessons*. Longmans, Green & Co. 1917.

6   Shephard, B. *Headhunters: the pioneers of neuroscience*. Vintage. 2014. p194.

7   Elliot Smith & Pear, op. cit.

8   MHFYN p1.

Chapter 11. LIFE IN A COLD CLIMATE

1   *The Sun*. 3 March 1932.

2   Birtles, B. 'Marcel Aurousseau: poetry, people, and places'. *Meanjin* 29. December 1968.

3   *The Sun*, op. cit.

4   *The Sun*. 10 March 1932.

5   Morison, P. *J. T. Wilson and the Fraternity of Duckmaloi*. Rodopi. 1997. p88.

6   *The Argus*. 3 September 1935.

7   Zuckerkandl, E. *Proceedings of the Anatomical Society of Great Britain and Ireland*. November 1931.

8   MHFYN p117.

9   Shine, R. 'Evolution of an Evolutionary Hypothesis: a history of changing ideas about the adaptive significance of viviparity in reptiles'. *Journal of Herpetology* 48(2). June 2014. pp147–61.

10 Weekes, H.C. 'A Review of Placentation among Reptiles with Particular Regard to the Function and Evolution of the Placenta'. *Journal of Zoology* 105(3). September 1935.

11 Rheubert, J.L. et al. *Reproductive Biology and Phylogeny of Lizards and Tuatara*. CRC Press. 2015. p530.

Chapter 12. THE SONG OF BETH

1 'Our History'. Sydney Conservatorium of Music. http://music. sydney.edu.au/about/history/

2 *Australian Town and Country Journal*. 17 October 1906.

3 *The Great Southern Herald*. 27 March 1912.

4 *The Sydney Morning Herald*. October 1906.

5 *The Sun*. 4 January 1922. p8.

6 *The Sunday Sun*. 3 October 1909. p12.

7 *The Sydney Morning Herald*. 5 December 1921.

8 *The Mudgee Guardian*. 26 April 1928. p9.

9 Murray, L. *Killing the Black Dog*. Black Inc. 2009. p7.

10 *Daily News* (Perth). 3 June 1935. p4.

11 *The Sydney Morning Herald*. 4 January 1936.

12 *The Sydney Morning Herald*. 1 August 1936.

13 *The Sydney Morning Herald*. 6 January 1936.

14 *Truth*. 21 June 1936.

15 *Newsletter* no. 6. 1937.

16 *The Sydney Morning Herald*. 21 January 1937.

Chapter 13. DR WEEKES' EUROPEAN TRAVEL ADVICE BUREAU

1 *The Advertiser* (Adelaide). 18 April 1939. p6.

2 Letter from Brian Weekes to his daughter Barbara Weekes, c. August/ September 1985.

3 *The Australian Women's Weekly*. 18 December 1937. p25.

4 Souter, G. *Company of Heralds*. Melbourne University Press. 1981. p625.

5 *The Advertiser*. 18 April 1939.

6 A documentary, *Deception by Design*, was made on this untold story in 2011.

7 *The Sporting Globe*. 17 April 1943.

Chapter 14. THE WORLD AT WAR

1 Oral history. National Library of Australia. Recorded by Hazel de Berg, 30 June 1977.

Chapter 15. DR WEEKES, REDUX

1 *The Sydney Morning Herald*. 2 December 1945.
2 Baker, R. (ed.) *Panic Disorder: theory, research, and therapy*. Wiley. 1989. p317.
3 Letter from Manuel D Zane to the Honours Secretariat, Government House, Canberra, Australia. 21 May 1990.
4 Tinbergen, N. 'Ethology and Stress Diseases'. Nobel Lecture. 12 December 1973.
5 TLHFYN p8.
6 ibid. pp1–2.
7 *Truth*. 27 September 1953.
8 ibid.

Chapter 16. THE HOUSE OF WOMEN

1 Oral history. National Library of Australia. Recorded by Hazel de Berg, 30 June 1977.
2 MHFYN p68.
3 Papers filed to the Supreme Court of New South Wales. Equity division. As stated of Hazel Claire Weekes deceased in the Family Provision Act 1982. Plaintiff Penelope Noel Weekes defendant Elizabeth Muir Louez.

Chapter 17. THE BIRTH OF A BOOK

1 TLHFYN p91.
2 *The Australian Women's Weekly*. 23 August 1978.

3   Roe, J. *Her Brilliant Career: the life of Stella Miles Franklin*. Belknap Press. 2009.

4   P.R. Stephensen papers. Mitchell Library, State Library of NSW.

5   Munro, C. *Wild Man of Letters: the story of P.R. Stephensen*. Melbourne University Press. 1984. p264.

6   ibid. p265.

7   Angus & Robertson collection. State Library of NSW.

8   Munro, op. cit. p265.

9   *The New York Times*. 24 February 1988.

10 Munro, op. cit. p270.

11 P.R. Stephensen papers, op. cit.

Chapter 18. SELF HELP FOR YOUR NERVES

1   *The Australian Women's Weekly*. 23 August 1979.

2   Letter to Robert DuPont. 4 April 1989.

3   *The Australian Women's Weekly*, op. cit.

4   Norman, A. 'Domestic Goddess to Sex Kitten: women's roles through *The Weekly*'. http://www.opus.org.au/articles/domestic-goddess-sex-kitten/

5   SHFYN p31.

6   'Mindfulness in Everyday Life'. Black Dog Institute. https://www.blackdoginstitute.org.au/docs/default-source/psychological-toolkit/7-mindfulnessineverydaylife-(with-gp-notes).pdf

7   PFNS p116.

8   SHFYN p3.

9   SETOA p24.

10 SHFYN p172.

11 ibid.

12 Letter from Robert DuPont to the Secretary of the Order of Australia. 31 May 1990.

13 PFNS p184.

14 Freeman, A. et al. *Clinical Applications of Cognitive Therapy*, 2nd ed. Springer. 2004. p150.

Chapter 19. UNSCIENTIFIC SCIENCE

1 O'Toole, G.B. *The Case against Evolution*. Macmillan. 1925. p37.
2 Ebert, A. & Bär, K-J. 'Emil Kraepelin: a pioneer of scientific understanding of psychiatry and psychopharmacology'. *Indian Journal of Psychiatry* 52(2). 2010.
3 McDougall, W. 'Fundamentals of Psychology: behaviourism explained'. 1929. http://psychclassics.yorku.ca/Watson/Battle/macdougall.htm [sic]
4 McLeod, S.A. 'Behaviourist Approach'. 2017. https://www.simplypsychology.org/behaviorism.html
5 Jackson, M. *The Age of Stress: science and the search for stability*. Oxford University Press. 2013. p2.
6 Valenstein, E.S. *The War of the Soups and the Sparks: the discovery of neurotransmitters and the dispute over how nerves communicate*. Columbia University Press. 2012.
7 Hollon, S.D. & DiGiuseppe, R. 'Cognitive Theories of Psychotherapy' in Norcross, J.C. et al. (eds) *History of Psychotherapy: continuity and change*, 2nd ed. American Psychological Association. 2010.
8 Ellis, A. 'Discomfort Anxiety: a new cognitive-behavioural construct, part I'. *Journal of Rational-Emotive and Cognitive-Behaviour Therapy* 21(3/4). Winter 2003.

Chapter 20. GETTING A GRIP ON THE MARKET

1 *The Australian Women's Weekly*. 26 December 1962. © Bauer Media Pty Limited.
2 Letter to Robert DuPont. 1989.

3   'Basics'. The Morita School of Japanese Psychology.
    http://www.moritaschool.com/read-me/

4   Watanabe, N. & Machleidt, W. 'Morita therapy: a Japanese method for
    treating neurotic anxiety syndrome'. *Der Nervenarzt* 74(11). November
    2003. pp1020–4.

5   Munro, C. *Wild Man of Letters: the story of P.R. Stephensen.*
    Melbourne University Press. 1984.

6   Angus & Robertson collection. State Library of NSW.

7   ibid. 19 May 1966.

8   ibid.

9   Letter (name and country withheld). 3 July 1965.

10 Angus & Robertson collection, op. cit.

Chapter 21. A SECOND HOME

1   TLHFYN p89.

Chapter 22. BAD BUSINESS

1   Letter to Robert DuPont. 15 January 1989.

2   Interview with Paddy Feeney. *Living with One's Fears.* BBC. 16
    February 1969.

3   'Anxiety-Ridden Housebound Women Must Learn Not to Fight Their
    Fears'. AP Newspapers. 28 July 1969.

4   ibid.

5   Weekes, C. *Pass Through Panic.* Audio.

6   'Learn How Not to Fight Fear'. *The San Francisco Examiner.* 10 August
    1969.

7   LeDoux, J. *Anxious: the modern mind in the age of anxiety* (UK edition).
    Oneworld. 2015. p26.

8   Graham, V. *If I Made It, So Can You.* Bantam. 1978. p2.

9   Letter to Robert DuPont. 1988.

10 *The Indianapolis News*. 14 November 1979.

11 Yianitsas, Y. 'A Personal Message from Jack Yianitsas.' n.d.

12 Letter from Jack Yianitsas to J.S. O'Connor Harris and co-barristers and solicitors. 25 April 1996.

Chapter 23. PEACE FROM AGORAPHOBIA

1   *Statesman Journal*. 20 July 1969.

2   *The Australian Women's Weekly*. 22 November 1972.

3   ibid.

4   *The Pensacola News Journal*. 27 July 1969. p48.

5   *Los Angeles Times*. 24 July 1969.

6   Barlow, D. https://www.youtube.com/watch?v=aqPhLlY8RLg

7   Barlow, D. https://www.youtube.com/watch?v=HHjnG5fFPYg

8   PFNS p14.

9   *Los Angeles Times*. 27 April 1972. p106.

10 Stott, C. 'The Permanent Prisoners'. *The Guardian*. 25 August 1972.

11 'Terror of Open Spaces'. *The Sunday Times*. 10 June 1973.

12 Weekes, C. 'A Practical Treatment of Agoraphobia'. *British Medical Journal* 2(5864). 26 May 1973. pp469–71.

13 'Advice Columnist Ann Landers Dead at 83'. *Chicago Tribune*. 22 June 2002.

14 *The Evening Review*. 30 July 1976.

15 *Press-Telegram*. 10 June 1973. p77.

16 *The Pittsburgh Press*. 24 April 1970. p13.

17 *The Daily Tribune*. 2 August 1969. p3.

Chapter 24. A PIONEER OF FEAR

1   LeDoux, J. 'Facing Fear'. https://www.youtube.com/watch?v=UbqoLdd1wpY

2 Ressler, K.R. quoted in LeDoux, J. *Anxious: the modern mind in the age of anxiety* (UK edition). Oneworld. 2015.

3 LeDoux, J. & Pine, D.S. 'Using Neuroscience to Help Understand Fear and Anxiety: a two-system framework'. *The American Journal of Psychiatry* 173(11). November 2016.

4 ibid.

5 LeDoux. *Anxious*, op. cit. p177.

6 Schore, A.N. *The Science of the Art of Psychotherapy*. W.W. Norton & Co. 2011.

7 LeDoux. 'Facing Fear', op. cit.

8 Barrett, L.F. https://www.youtube.com/watch?v=kY6mCVCubjI

9 PFNS p60.

10 Sapolsky, R. *Behave: the biology of humans at our best and worst*. Bodley Head. 2017. p153.

11 LeDoux. *Anxious*, op. cit. p317.

Chapter 25. LIVING IN TWO WORLDS

1 *The Argus*. 22 August 1976.

Chapter 26. THE SOULMATE

1 *The Baltimore Sun*. 26 December 1976.

2 SETOA p4.

3 ibid. p3.

4 ibid.

5 Barlow, D. http://podbay.fm/show/218827921/e/1200513360

6 Barlow, D. https://www.youtube.com/watch?v=HHjnG5fFPYg

7 SETOA p125.

8 'Tom Snyder, Pioneer of Late-Night Television, Dies at 71'. *The New York Times*. 31 July 2007.

9   Sarpa, J.J. 'A Historical Study of Mental Health Programming in Commercial and Public Television from 1975 to 1980'. Dissertation. 1985.

10 SETOA p29.

11 MHFYN.

12 *The New York Times Magazine*. December 1977.

13 *The Daily*. 4 January 1979.

14 'Dr Claire Weekes: healer of shattered nerves'. *The Australian Women's Weekly*. 23 August 1978.

15 ibid.

Chapter 27. VINDICATION

1   Decker, H. *The Making of DSM-III*. Oxford University Press. 2013.

2   ibid.

3   SETOA p24.

4   *The New York Times*. 31 October 1991.

5   Pols, H. & Oak, S. 'War & Military Health: the US psychiatric response in the 20th century'. *American Journal of Public Health* 97(12). December 2007. pp2132–42.

6   SHFYN p65.

7   Schwartz, T.L. & Petersen, T. (eds) *Depression: treatment strategies and management*. CRC Press. 2016. p308.

8   MHFYN p117.

Chapter 28. OLD AGE

1   Marks, I.M. *Fears, Phobias, and Rituals: panic, anxiety, and their disorders*. Oxford University Press. 1987. p338.

2   Letter from Robert DuPont to the Secretary of the Order of Australia. 31 May 1990.

3   MHFYN p68.

4   ibid. p84.

5   ibid. p116.

6   TLHFYN p98.

Chapter 29. THE BBC AND A BLIZZARD OF LETTERS

1   Letter from Anne Turner. 13 May 1998.

Chapter 30. THE SOUND OF CLOSING DOORS

1   Letter from Weekes' agent Al Zuckerman. 26 March 1986.

2   Letter from Brian Weekes to his daughter Barbara Weekes, c. August/
     September 1985.

Chapter 32. EYES ON THE PRIZE

1   Letter to Robert DuPont. 15 January 1989.

Chapter 33. THE NOBEL NOMINATION

1   Letter to Robert DuPont. 31 January 1989.

2   Baker, R. *Understanding Panic Attacks and Overcoming Fear*, 3rd ed. Lion
     Books. 2011.

Chapter 34. FINAL DAYS

1   MHFYN p85.

Epilogue: WHAT LIVES ON

1   Fassaie, S. *Rising from the Shadows: revolution, war, and the journey that
     made me*. Richmond Press. 2015.

Acknowledgements

1   LeDoux, J. *Anxious: the modern mind in the age of anxiety* (UK edition). Oneworld. 2015.

2   Baker, R. (ed.) *Panic Disorder: theory, research, and therapy*. Wiley. 1989.

Index